MW01249014

HEALING

IN

HALACHAH

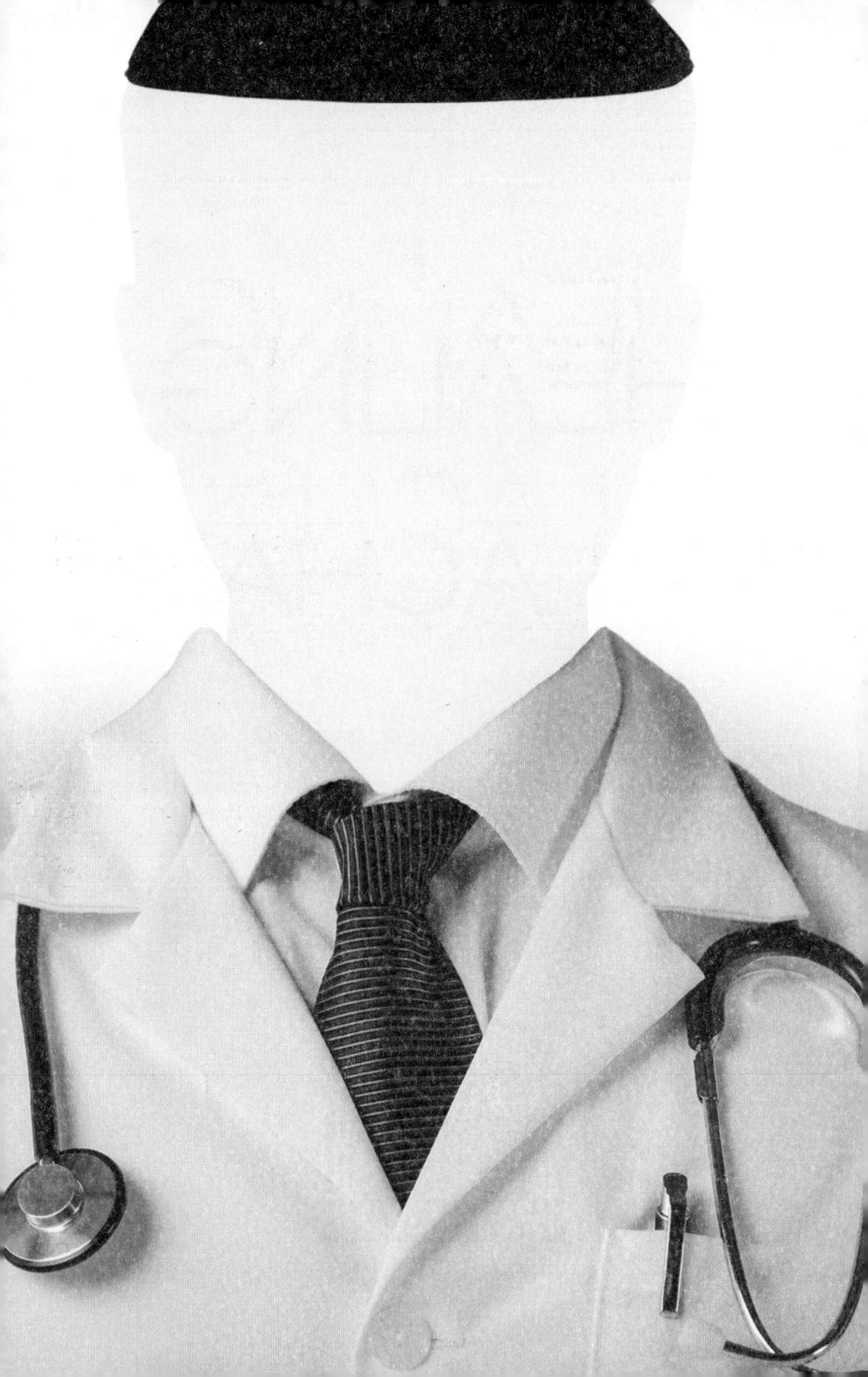

HEALING IN HALACHAH

RABBI MICHA A. COHN

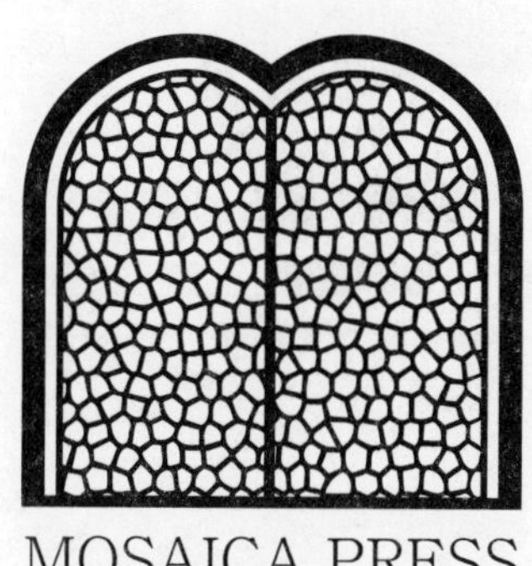

MOSAICA PRESS

Mosaica Press, Inc.

Designed and typeset by Rayzel Broyde

ISBN-10: 1-937887-79-0

ISBN-13: 978-1-937887-79-7

Published and distributed by:

Mosaica Press, Inc.

www.mosaicapress.com

info@mosaicapress.com

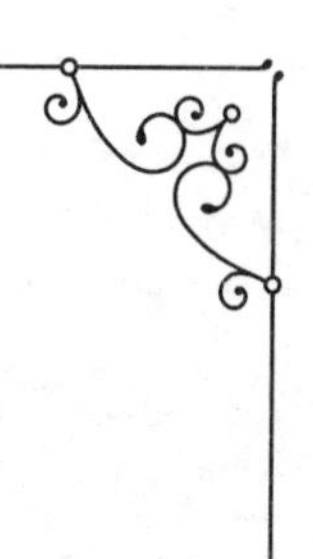

This *sefer* is dedicated *l'zechus refuah sheleimah* for

Shoshana bas Chaya Leah

BY DRS. JAY AND MELISSA BERNSTEIN AND FAMILY

ולעילוי נשמת

HaGaon Rav Yisroel Belsky, zt"l

Who reviewed this work but was *niftar* before he could give his written *haskamah*

BY A TALMID

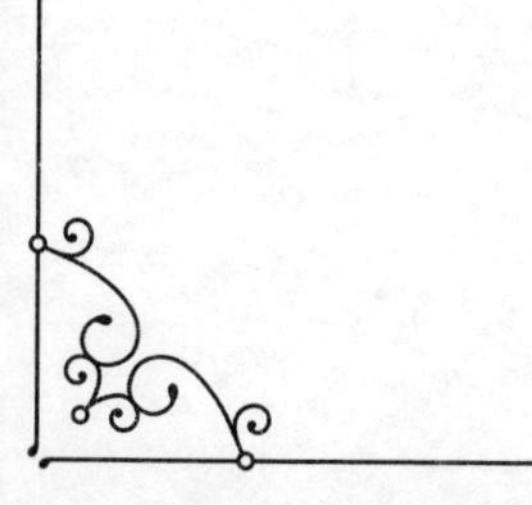

בס"ד

שמואל קמנצקי
Rabbi S. Kamenetsky

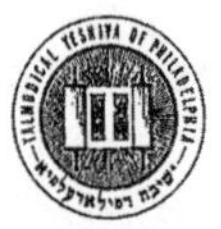

2018 Upland Way
Philadelphia, PA 19131

Home: 215-473-2798
Study: 215-473-1212

בס"ד ע' פ' ויקהל תשע"ו

ראיתי הסכמת הרה"ג ר' יעקב אפרים פארבער
בארה"ב ומו"ה שליט"א על הספר אשר עומד הר"ר מנחם
כהן שליט"א להוציא לאור.

הדברים דבחירות ובחירות בלשון שהיא מובנת
לכל אחד על נכון, ונלקטו הדברים מספרים חשובים
ראשונים ואחרונים. והוא יש צורך גדול לכך.

הנני מאחל שיזכה ה' בידו וזכות ויזכה להפיץ
מעיינותיו חוצה. והשי"ת יתן שיתעוררו לעסוק בתורה
ולהפיצה.

בכבוד וברכה
שמואל קמנצקי

Yaakov E. Forchheimer
604 Sixth Street
Lakewood, N.J. 08701
(732) 364-4919

יעקב אפרים הכהן פארכהיימער
מו"ץ בק"ק
לייקוואוד יצ"ו

בס"ד

הנה ראיתי הקונטרס שחבר ידידי מוה"ר מיכה הכהן שליט"א שכולל שאלות נחוצות בעניני רפואה והמסתעף מזה, והביא צדדי השאלה ודעות הפוסקים בזה ואיך לנהוג למעשה.

דבר גדול עשה בישראל להורות הדרך ילכו בה, ולא יהיו הענינים החמורים האלו מסורים ביד כל אחד להכריע כדעתו מה לעשות.

ויש גם כן תועלת גדולה לתלמידי חכמים ליקט המציאות של הדברים והמקורות בפוסקים להשאלות האלו לסייעם לפסוק הלכה על בוריה.

ומה שכתב אודות הנהגת מכוניות ודאי דבר נחוץ הוא למאד, ויש בזה גם משום חילול ה' ר"ל כנודע.

לכן ראוי להדפיס הקונטרס הזה ולהפיצו בישראל לזכות את הרבים.

יזכה הרב המחבר שליט"א לישב באהלה של תורה כל ימיו ולהיות ממרביצי התורה ומזכי הרבים.

על זה באתי על החתום יום ג' לס' פסח וישב יו"ט לחג רגלי תשס"ו

יעקב אפרים הכהן פארכהיימער

בע"ה

RABBI ARYEH MALKIEL KOTLER
BETH MEDRASH GOVOHA
LAKEWOOD, N.J. 08701

ארי' מלכיאל קוטלר
בית מדרש גבוה
לייקוואוד, נ. דז.

כ"ב אדר א' תשע"ו

בהתהלכך תנחה אותך בשכבך תשמור עליך והקיצות היא תשיחך (משלי ו' כב')

הפסוק כולל כל חלקי החיים הלכות החיים שהתורה מנחה דרכיה והתורה מנחה הדרך של כל פסיעה שהאדם הולך בה אם ללכת ולאן וכו' וכו', וגם כשכבו הרי הוא דבוק בהתורה עד כדי שגם שינתו אינו נהפסק בלימודו ועד כדי שבהקיצו הרי ממש כאמצע לימודו והשיחה במילא שלו היא בתורה, וכל ענין בחיי האדם בכל התורה היא המנחה והמורה דרך לאותה הענין ובפרט גם ענייני רפואה של כל צער וסבל התורה אומרת איך להתנהג

אפריון נמטיה למע"כ ידידי התה"ג ר' מיכה כהן שליט"א מחשובי האברכים פה בישיבתנו הק', לן בעומקה של הלכה ושקלא וטריא כינס בעמל התורה ולאוסופי שמעתא להלכתא, ועכשיו מוציא לאור עולם ספר בשפה המדוברת בענין הנהגת הרפואה על הלכה אשר ליקט ערך וסידר וגיבר ולבן דברי גדולי הרבנים בעניינים חמורים אלו ואף שלא השגתי לעיין עליו להיות שר המסכים על הלכות למעשה, ובפרט בהיות ערכו הרם בתורה, ונאמנים עלי דברי הגאונים הפוסקים שליט"א הגאון ר' יונתן אברהם הכהן שליט"א ועוד גדולי הפוסקים בדבר הלכה למעשה, והספר הזה בודאי לתועלת ללומדים ומעיינים בסוגיות אלו וגם לשואל ולהאיר את ענינים אלו ויה"ר שיתקבלו דבריו בבי מדרשא, עוד יוסיף כהנה וכהנה לזכות לאור ספרים, ולהמשיך עבודתו בקודש ללון בעומקה של הלכה להגדיל תורה ולהאדירה.

הכותב לכבוד התורה ולומדיה
אריה מלכיאל קוטלר
בא"א מו"ר הגר"ש זצוק"ל

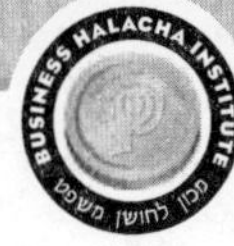

BAIS HORA'AH EITZ CHAIM
בית הוראה עץ חיים

RAV CHAIM KOHN, *Dean*
הרב חיים קאהן שליט"א, אב"ד

בס"ד

מוצש"ק פ' ויקהל תשע"ו

לכבוד ידידי היקר הרה"ג ר' מיכה כהן שליט"א

הודעתני שאתה עומד להדפיס את השיעורים שנתת בעניני רפואה ובמשך הזמן נקבצו יחד לכדי ספר שלם. המאמרים מצטיינים בבהירות ההסבר והיקף הנושא, ואינו פלא שמצאו מאוד חן בעיני שומעי וקוראי לקחך.

ובכן גם אני מצטרף בשמחה לשאר המברכים שתמשיך בהצלחה בעבודת הקודש, ללמוד וללמד לשמור ולשעות.

ידידך החפץ בהצלחתך

חיים קאהן

1937 OCEAN AVENUE | BROOKLYN, NEW YORK 11230 | 718.233.3845 | 718.705.5429 FAX | ASK@BUSINESSHALACHA.COM

TABLE OF CONTENTS

ACKNOWLEDGMENTS

The book you are holding wasn't born overnight. It is actually an adaptation of nearly a hundred email posts from The Medical Halachah Email for Professionals that I started in 2011. I am humbled by the hundreds of medical and mental health professionals who took interest in my work. I am greatly indebted to you for your valuable questions and comments.

My journey into medical halachah goes back further. I would like to take this opportunity to thank the many people who helped me along the way.

More than ten years ago, while learning in Beth Medrash Govoha, I began regularly attending the *shiurim* of Rabbi Dovid Feinstein *shlit"a* in Mesivta Tifereth Jerusalem. The Rosh Yeshiva, *hanhalah*, and *talmidim* of MTJ have been ever so gracious to me. The Rosh Yeshiva is an address for the most complex halachic questions from around the world. Being in his presence has had a profound impact on me. I have also had the opportunity to benefit from another of Rabbi Moshe Feinstein's great *talmidim*, Rabbi Elimelech Bluth *shlit"a*.

Around the same time I began interning under Rabbi Shlomo Stern, the Debretzener Rav of Boro Park and the Beis Hora'ah of Karlsberg under the leadership of Rabbi Yechezkel Roth *shlit"a*. Rabbi Roth is one of the greatest *poskim* in the Chassidic world today. The time I spent sitting at his side while throngs of people presented their questions is priceless. I am also indebted to Rabbi Avrohom Yehoshua Heshel Bick, Rav of Kahal Mezibuz in Boro Park, for the time and warmth he has shown me.

Back in Lakewood I have been equally blessed. For the past several years I have had the opportunity to assist Rabbi Shmuel Meir Katz, senior *posek* for Beth Medrash Govoha as a member of his Beis Hora'ah. Rabbi Katz's tremendous knowledge in the intricacies of so many areas of halachah has been a great resource for me.

Around seven years ago I began interning at the Beis Din of Philadelphia under Rabbi Ahron Felder *zt"l* and Rabbi Dov Brisman *shlit"a*. Rabbi Felder was one of the greatest *talmidim* of Rabbi Moshe Feinstein and a scion of rabbinic lineage. After interning at the Beis Din for a few years, he graciously gave me a full *semichah*. Subsequently, we worked together to publish his notes from the fourteen years he spent at Reb Moshe's side. Rabbi Felder's eyesight was failing and I did the writing and helped look up the sources. Notwithstanding his physical limitations, Rabbi Felder's spirit was sharp, robust, and full of life. Sadly, he passed away suddenly at the age of seventy. I still long to call him again and often reach for the phone when a complex question arises. He always encouraged me to write and publish. I hope this work is a source of *nachas* for him and the Rebbitzen *shetichyeh*. *Yehi zichro baruch*.

I cannot thank enough Rabbi Shalom Kamenetsky, Rosh Yeshivah of the Philadelphia Yeshivah. He has been there for me since the start of this project and at every step along the way. His advice and encouragement have been indispensable.

The encouragement of my longtime rebbe, Rabbi Mordechai Respler, Rosh Yeshivah of Mesivta of Long Beach, and Rabbi Elya Brudny, Rosh Yeshivas Mir, have been priceless.

I am deeply indebted to Rabbi Chaim Kohn, Dean of the Business Halachah Institute. It has been a great privilege to write for such an important institution. Rabbi Kohn's breadth of halachah and understanding of the workings of the world is profound. He has always been a valuable source of advice and encouragement for the medical halachah email.

There are a number of people who have helped me gain a better understanding of medicine and the challenges observant professionals face. Dr. Binyamin Sokol, a pioneer in the field of Jewish medical ethics and a former ethics committee member in Chicago, shared with me the lessons on medical ethics he presented to medical students in Chicago. Dr. Elliot Frank of Jersey Shore University Medical Center literally opened the hospital to me. He allowed me to participate (I.D. in all!) as a medical student in morning reports and other trainings.

As a Bostonian, I have been blessed with close relationships with some superb physicians who exemplify a beautiful combination of *ehrlichkeit* and professionalism. Dr. Chuna Chaim Lebowitz has been a great resource for me on End of Life Issues. Dr. Boruch Feinberg spent hours with me in his office going through the intricacies of gynecology and obstetrics. Drs. Yaakov and Sandra Weinreb and Dr. Robby Lowenstein have been great friends and teachers in their respective fields. Robby, without you I don't know if this project would have gotten off the ground! Dr. Klompas, an expert in infectious disease, has always been willing to discuss my questions.

I have always been fascinated with mental health. Dr. Shmuel Millman and Dr. David Rosmarin have been great friends and teachers. Much of the section in this book on mental health is based on Dr. Rosmarin's questions. I would also like to thank Rabbi Moshe Markowitz MSW of Baltimore for sharing with me his interest in the interface between Torah and personality disorders.

I would like to thank our friends Yair and Esty Stern for the opportunity to give *shiurim* for physician's assistants and nurse practitioners in their home. The *shiurim* have been a great experience for me.

Thank you to my longtime *chavrusa*, Rabbi Yaakov Shulman, for plumbing the depths of so many intricate *sugyos* with me.

I would like to thank Beth Medrash Govoha, which has provided me a first-class environment to grow in Torah scholarship for the last twelve years. I would like to thank my alma mater, the Mesivta of Long Beach, *hanhalah*, and esteemed Rosh Yeshivah, Rabbi Yitzchok Feigelstock. I am deeply grateful to Rabbi Shimon Alster, Rosh Yeshivah of Cliffwood Yeshiva.

Closer to home, I am forever indebted to my dear parents Rabbi

Dovid and Chaya Sarah Cohn of Boston and most recently of Hollywood, Florida. The imprint of their exemplary *chinuch*, love, and encouragement is etched in every page of this book. I hope it gives them much *nachas*. Thank you to my dear in-laws, Rabbi Boruch and Shaindy Stark for being so supportive of everything that I do and to my wonderful brothers and sisters-in-law for being such an important part of my life. Thank you to my dear brother Rabbi Avrohom, my good friend and confidant, and his wonderful family. The work all of you do to spread Torah in Phoenix, Arizona, is an inspiration. Most of all, I would like to thank my wife Gitty, my partner in every way, and our children Yaakov Mordechai and Tziporah Leah, for being the light of our lives.

I would like to express my appreciation to all the places that give me the opportunity to teach Torah on a regular basis. Much of my day is spent teaching halachah to the students of Yeshiva Meor HaTalmud in Lakewood, New Jersey. The shining faces and inquisitive minds of the *talmidim* brighten my days. Thank you to Mr. Ezra and Shuly Klein of Agra DePirka and to all the participants. It is a privilege to teach Torah to such a distinguished group of people. Thank you to the participants of the Sunday morning *kollel* of Kahal Daas Kedoshim of Coventry Square. Those mornings are a highlight of my week.

The idea of adapting the emails into a book was in the back of my mind for a long time. However, it just sat there. Where to begin with such a project? Thank you to Rabbi Yaacov Haber, Rabbi Doron Kornbluth, Tzvi, and Yehoshua Haber of Mosaica Press for reaching out to me. Working with you on this project has been a great experience. A special thanks to Rabbi Kornbluth, the editor of this project, who has been there for me at every step of the way.

I would like to thank Rabbi Yaakov Forchheimer, senior *posek* at Beth Medrash Govoha and Rav of Kahal Sheiris Adas Yisroel, for taking the time from his extremely busy schedule to review and comment on every page of this work.

I am grateful to Rabbi Yisroel Belsky, *zt"l*, Rosh Yeshivas Torah Vodaath, for reviewing this work and for sharing with me his thoughts and encouragement. Sadly, he was taken from us before he could grace this work with his written *haskamah*. *Yehi zichro baruch*.

Most importantly, I would like to thank you, the reader, for taking the time and interest to read this book.

Micha A. Cohn
Cheshvan 5776

INTRODUCTION

This book is not a practical guide to medical halachah. It is an overview of the complex issues that need to be addressed before arriving at a decision. I hope it will help patients, their caregivers, and those who practice medicine present their questions to a competent halachic authority with more clarity.

A few points on the study of halachah: the study of halachah really has two components. The learning of halachah begins with the study of the classic sources in the Talmud, Rishonim, *Shulchan Aruch* with its commentaries, and important rabbinic responsa, with its differing opinions. However, taking all the opinions into consideration and formulating a conclusion is a study unto itself. The art of halachic decision making is called *hora'ah*, which comes from the word *lehoros* — to show. It shows a path between the plethora of sources, ideas, and opinions.

Halachic decision making is not a free-for-all. It has a specific methodology. While rabbis often differ in their conclusions, their decision-making process must follow one of three basic methods. Rabbi Moshe Isserles, the Rema, writes: "When there is a difference of opinion, a rabbi should not say 'I will rule according to whom I like...' if he does so, it is not a true ruling."[1] The Rema then gives three methods a rabbi could use to arrive at a decision. 1. If he is a great scholar he can prove which opinion is correct and arrive at his own conclusion. 2. He can follow the general rule that when there is a doubt or difference of opinion

1 *Shulchan Aruch*, Choshen Mishpat 25:2.

concerning a Torah prohibition one must be stringent. However, if it is a rabbinic prohibition one may be lenient. Likewise, he may follow the majority opinion.[2] 3. If there is an accepted custom to follow a specific opinion, it may be followed even if it is a minority opinion.[3]

This work does not seek to decide the questions that are discussed. Rather, the various opinions are presented and the different aspects of the issue at hand are weighed. Often we try to determine if the question is of Torah or rabbinic nature. While rabbinic prohibitions are an indispensable part of Judaism, the Sages often allowed us to be more lenient when the question is of rabbinic nature. Understanding the underlying principles and discussions will help the reader gain a sense for what types of situations pose serious halachic challenges and which situations do not. For a final decision in a specific situation, the guidance of a competent *posek* is indispensable.

A few additional points: Halachah is comprised of two basic bodies of literature: the classic codes with their commentaries, and rabbinic responsa. The codes focus on understanding the foundations and principles of the halachah. The responsa address how rabbis actually formulated their decisions in real-life situations. In this work, we will draw greatly from rabbinic responsa spanning nearly a thousand years.

When citing a source or translating a quotation, I took the liberty to explain it according to my understanding of its meaning, not necessarily the literal translation. I encourage you to look up the sources yourself. My work is only intended as a springboard for further study.

I hope this work will provide food for thought and a window into the great discussions found in halachic literature. I hope it will promote a better appreciation for the halachic decision-making process and will share the beauty of how age-old halachic sources address the most cutting-edge medical technology. I hope this book will help people ask better questions that will enable them to receive better answers.

---

2 The Shach writes that in extenuating circumstances, it is sometimes permitted to follow a minority opinion.

3 The Pri Chadash (Hilchos Pesach) writes that the reason why Sephardic Jews customarily follow the opinions of the Rambam, Ramban, and Rashba, whereas Ashkenazim follow the opinions of Tosfos, is because each community accepted them as their teachers.

Section I:
SHABBOS

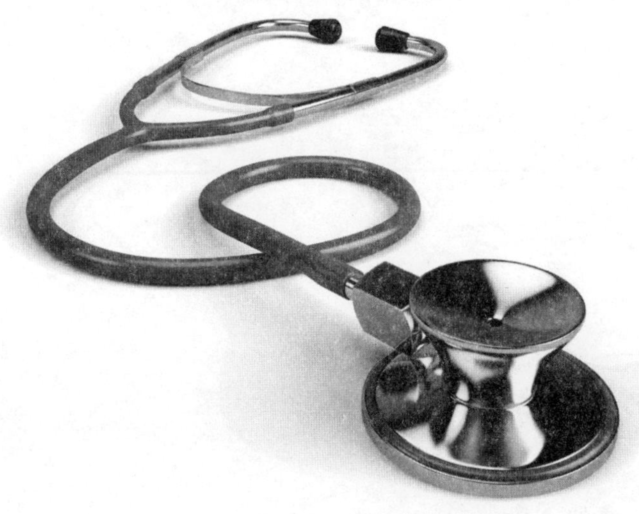

PIKUACH NEFESH ISSUES

Testing Blood Sugar on Shabbos

Q: Is it permitted to test blood sugar on Shabbos? How should a diabetic approach this issue?

A: It would seem that drawing blood for the purpose of using it for a test is a Torah prohibition. Unlike bleeding caused inadvertently during an injection, here the blood is being used for something constructive.

On the other hand, diabetes is a clear life-threatening ailment that needs to be managed. Therefore, routine testing should be permitted as *pikuach nefesh*. The remaining question is how careful must one be in order to not test more than what is absolutely necessary.

Several approaches should be mentioned:

- Interestingly, there is an important opinion of the Rambam that once a person is classified as dangerously ill, all forms of care are permitted on Shabbos, even if it is just for the person's comfort.[4]

4 *Shabbos* 2:1; *Shulchan Aruch*, Orach Chaim 328:4, *Mishnah Berurah* 14.

- Other opinions disagree and maintain that only treatment that is necessary to preserve life is permitted on Shabbos.[5]
- There is an interesting middle approach that the disagreement is only regarding things that are not part of the care of the life-threatening ailment. However, medical care that is part of managing the life-threatening illness, even when it does not seem crucial, is still permissible because it could affect the illness in an indirect way.[6]

Based on these sources, it seems that standard protocol should always be followed, unless it is absolutely clear that postponing the blood sugar test will not have any effect on the ailment. We will expand on these ideas in our next discussion.

Desecrating Shabbos for the Nonessential Care of a Seriously Ill Patient

Q: When caring for a patient who has a dangerous ailment (*choleh sheyeish bo sakanah*), is desecrating Shabbos only permitted for elements of the care that are absolutely necessary, or even for general care and comfort?

A: There is an important discussion about the scope of the permission to desecrate Shabbos for a dangerously ill patient. Here are some important points:

5 See *Mishnah Berurah* ibid.

6 See *Avnei Nezer*, Orach Chaim 453.

The Basic Sources

The *Shulchan Aruch* writes, quoting the Rambam, that for a dangerous internal wound, "we do ***everything*** that is normally done for it during the week."[7] The Maggid Mishnah understands the broad wording of the Rambam to even permit aspects of the care that there is no risk to withhold. However, Rashi, Rashba, and other Rishonim write clearly that a Torah prohibition may only be done for aspects of the care that are life-threatening.

The *Mishnah Berurah* points out that many Rishonim do not permit desecrating Shabbos for non-*pikuach nefesh* aspects of care.[8] Therefore, a Torah prohibition should not be transgressed if it is clear that withholding the care will not have an adverse effect on the patient's condition. In a similar vein, the Shulchan Aruch HaRav brings both opinions and concludes that it is better to have a non-Jew do the *melachah*.[9] However, if it is not possible, the first opinion may be relied upon but recommends avoiding a Torah prohibition.

Hutra or Dechuya?

Many later commentaries understand that this question is connected to a fundamental question about the concept of *pikuach nefesh*. When *pikuach nefesh* allows desecrating the Shabbos, does the prohibition becomes *hutra* — completely permitted — or only *dechuya* — pushed aside? If it is *hutra*, there is no reason to minimize how much *melachah* is done. However, if it is only *dechuya*, then desecrating Shabbos is only permitted for necessities.

The question of *hutra* or *dechuya* is discussed in the Rishonim. Rashi, Rashba, and Ran are of the opinion that Shabbos is only *dechuya*. However, Rabbi Ovadia Yosef points out that Tosfos, Maharam MeRuttenberg, Rosh, Mordechai, Tur, Rabeinu Yeshaya, and Tashbatz are all of the opinion that Shabbos is *hutra* for *pikuach nefesh*.[10] It is plausible that the *Shulchan Aruch* follows the approach of *hutra*. This would

---

7 Orach Chaim 328:4.

8 Biur Halachah on *Shulchan Aruch* ibid., s.v. *kol*; *Mishnah Berurah* 14.

9 328:4.

10 *Yechaveh Da'as* 4:30.5.

explain why the *Shulchan Aruch* used broad terms when permitting desecrating Shabbos for a seriously ill patient.

The Rambam's Position

An important consideration with applying the concepts of *hutra* and *dechuya* to our question about nonessential care is the position of the Rambam. The Rambam writes that Shabbos is desecrated for *all* care of a seriously ill patient. This implies that he holds that even nonessential care is permitted. It should follow that the Rambam takes the approach of *hutra*. However, he writes the exact opposite, saying that Shabbos is *dechuya* for *pikuach nefesh*!

Many commentators, including the great Rogochover Gaon, feel that the Rambam essentially holds that Shabbos is *hutra*. For various reasons they trivialize the wording of *dechuya* in the Rambam. However, the Radvaz did not follow this approach.

The Radvaz's Approach

Rabbi Dovid ben Zamra, the Radvaz, was the leader of Egyptian Jewry following the expulsion from Spain and an important authority on the Rambam. In his responsa, he was asked our question — whether Shabbos may be violated for nonessential care. He responded that some rabbis are lenient and some are strict, but "I would be from the lenient." At the same time, he writes that Shabbos is only *dechuya*.[11]

The Radvaz, however, does find a middle ground. He writes: "If there is no need at all, Shabbos should not be desecrated. Nonetheless, if there is somewhat of a need, it is permitted. Otherwise, this may cause them to be lax about giving essential care. While the possibility of this happening may be far-fetched, Shabbos may be desecrated for *pikuach nefesh* even if there are multiple doubts."

Simply put, the reason why the Radvaz permitted nonessential care was out of concern that once we start questioning what is really necessary, we could get into a hesitant attitude when caring for a patient on Shabbos, which could lead to real *pikuach nefesh*.

---

11 4:30.

The Avnei Nezer's Approach

The Avnei Nezer adds a whole new dimension to this discussion.[12] He redefines how risks are considered *pikuach nefesh*. Usually, we define care as *pikuach nefesh* if withholding it will directly put the patient in danger. The Avnei Nezer broadens this definition by asserting that although withholding the care will not cause a serious risk, it could cause a setback by weakening the patient and agitating the underlying illness.[13] He understands that putting the patient in greater risk of a setback is what is considered *pikuach nefesh*, although it is very indirect.[14]

The Meiri's Comments

The approach of the Avnei Nezer may also explain an apparent contradiction in the Meiri.[15] The Meiri writes that it is permitted to desecrate Shabbos for the sake of calming a woman after childbirth. The reason he gives is because her residual fear may put her in danger. Since he gives a reason for allowing Shabbos desecration, it implies that there is no broad leniency for nonessential care of a seriously ill patient. However, he also writes that any care that speeds up the healing process is permitted, even if the patient would not be in danger without it. This seems to assert that nonessential care is permitted.

Based on the Avnei Nezer, it would seem that the Meiri is only limiting care that is purely for comfort. However, care that aids in the healing process, which will ultimately take the patient out of the danger zone, is still considered *pikuach nefesh*.[16]

---

12 On Orach Chaim 453.

13 This is similar to the approach of Rabbi Chaim Soloveitchik, as cited by his son the Brisker Rav, *Chidushei HaGriz*, Hilchos Shvisas Assar.

14 This is an interesting point. Today medical professionals rely heavily on statistics that may not take into account factors like stress and other forms of discomfort, even though they could play a role in the general outcome but are difficult to prove.

15 Cited in Biur Halachah 328:4, s.v. *kol*.

16 Similarly, the Aruch HaShulchan understands that the wording of the Rambam that Shabbos is *dechuya* means that it is just not permitted entirely, and therefore anything that has a benefit to the healing process would certainly be permitted and not subject to scrutiny.

The Avnei Nezer's Conclusion

The Avnei Nezer acknowledges that his understanding of the Radvaz may be subject to disagreement. However, he lists the *Shulchan Aruch*, Dagul Merivavah, Karban Nesanel — "who was a great person" [his addition], and the Vilna Gaon who all seem to permit nonessential care. Therefore, he writes: "I am not worthy of deciding differently from the *Shulchan Aruch*, and if such a question would come before me, I would not be stringent about *pikuach nefesh*."

It is possible that the Avnei Nezer's conclusion does not contradict the opinions of the Biur Halachah and Shulchan Aruch HaRav mentioned above, who only permit violating a rabbinic prohibition for nonessential care. We first must consider why the Shulchan Aruch HaRav and Biur Halachah did not follow the rule of being lenient for *pikuach nefesh*. The answer is that since they were dealing with care that is completely unnecessary, there is no element of *pikuach nefesh* involved. As such, in the Avnei Nezer's case, where the care may have some impact on the patient's recovery, they may still consider it to be an issue of *pikuach nefesh*. Therefore, the Biur Halachah and Shulchan Aruch HaRav may agree that in these cases the general rule of being lenient for *pikuach nefesh* applies.

Conclusion

In conclusion, three levels of care for a seriously ill patient emerge from our discussion:

- Care that is clearly necessary in treating the dangerous ailment — this is unequivocally permitted on Shabbos even if it involves a Torah prohibition.
- Care that is solely for comfort — this is subject to a dispute. It is recommended to avoid transgressing a Torah prohibition, but it may be done through a non-Jew. A rabbinic prohibition is permitted.
- Care where there is no clear risk of life if withheld, but is standard protocol and affects the overall wellbeing of the patient or accelerates the healing process may fall into the first category

and is possibly permitted if it cannot be done through a non-Jew or in a form that is only rabbinic.

Segulos, Unconventional Remedies, and Pikuach Nefesh

Q: Is it permitted to transgress a prohibition like Shabbos or kashrus to perform a *segulah* or unconventional remedy in a life-threatening situation?

A: Here are some interesting points:

Rabbi Shlomo Kluger and the Rebbe of Belz

Around 150 years ago, a person was deathly ill on Shabbos and a *dayan* permitted desecrating the Shabbos in order to send a message to the great Rebbe of Belz, who was known as a miracle worker, to pray for the person. When Rabbi Shlomo Kluger, one of the leading halachic authorities of the time, heard about this ruling, he ordered the *dayan* to be fired for ruling incorrectly. The Tzemach Tzedek of Lubavitch, however, discusses this question in his responsa and rules otherwise.[17]

Much of this discussion focuses around the comments of the Rambam in his commentary on the Mishnah. There is a disagreement in the Mishnah about using a nonkosher remedy for the bite of a rabid dog. The Sages did not permit this remedy, despite this situation being one of *pikuach nefesh*. Rashi explains that although the physicians of the time used the remedy, it wasn't credible. According to some Rishonim, it wasn't a real remedy at all, but possibly a placebo. The Rambam, however,

17 See *Nishmas Avraham* on Orach Chaim 301:27, 328:2.

explains that the reason why it was prohibited is because it was not conventional medicine, rather a *segulah*, like an amulet, and not based on nature. He states that the concept of *pikuach nefesh* does not apply to supernatural remedies.

Rabbi Kluger in his responsa understands, based on the Rambam, that even if the miracle worker would have a 100 percent success rate, it is still prohibited to desecrate the Shabbos to seek him. This is because there is no leniency of *pikuach nefesh* for supernatural healing. The Maharsham cites Rabbi Kluger's opinion but concludes that if it would be so reliable, then the concern of the Rambam may not apply.

Rabbi Wosner on Homeopathy

Rabbi Shmuel Wosner, a contemporary halachic authority, discusses if the leniency of *pikuach nefesh* applies to alternative therapies like homeopathy.[18] In his discussion, he cites the Rambam and asks why *pikuach nefesh* doesn't override a Torah prohibition regardless of how the medicine works, natural or supernatural. He points out that a careful study of the Rambam would indicate that the Rambam's point was that these remedies were not tested and were not at all reliable. This was the primary reason why they are not permitted in a situation of *pikuach nefesh*. Based on this approach, Rabbi Wosner writes that alternative therapies can override Shabbos or kashrus in a situation of *pikuach nefesh* if there is some credible evidence that they work.

Conclusion

Natural remedies that are based on unconventional medicine need to have some level of credibility in order to apply the leniency of *pikuach nefesh*. *Segulos*, amulets, prayer, and other supernatural ways of healing, even if they are well established, may still not have the dispensation of *pikuach nefesh*.

---

18 *Shevet HaLevi* 5:55.

Desecrating Shabbos to Avoid Yichud Issues

Q: A patient is traveling to the hospital on Shabbos. Can an additional person come along for the sole purpose of being a *shomer* (guardian) to avoid *yichud* (forbidden seclusion) issues if it involves desecrating Shabbos? For example, traveling outside the *techum* or possibly causing the car to burn more gas?

A: We will begin with a discussion about a similar case from the 1800s and will then evaluate how it applies to our case.

Early Discussions

The Shem Aryeh was asked if an additional person could travel with a sick person on a wagon to avoid issues of *yichud*.[19] He analyzes the question in an interesting way. He starts off by stating that it is commonly known that all prohibitions are pushed aside in situations of *pikuach nefesh* except for the three cardinal sins of idolatry, immorality, and murder, which are considered *yaiharaig ve'al ya'avor* — die [lit. "killed"] rather than transgress. The Talmud in *Sanhedrin* teaches that even lesser forms of these sins have this similar stringency of *yaiharaig ve'al ya'avor*.[20] This concept is known as *abizraihu*.

Being that *yichud* is a safeguard from immorality, the Shem Aryeh questions if it has the status of *abizraihu*. If this is so, we have an interesting problem. The issue of *yichud* would prohibit the sick person from going in the wagon alone even at the expense of his life. As such, having a person go along would be considered *pikuach nefesh*. It would resolve the issue of *abizraihu* and would allow us to save the sick person's life. For this reason, *pikuach nefesh*

---

19 *Shem Aryeh*, cited in *Otzar HaPoskim*, Even HaEzer 22:1.

20 75a; see Shach, Yoreh Dei'ah 157:10.

would permit the extra person to go along in order to resolve the issue of *abizraihu*.

On the other hand, if *yichud* is not *abizraihu*, then it is permitted for the sake of *pikuach nefesh*. As such, it is not necessary for the additional person to desecrate the Shabbos to come along since *pikuach nefesh* overrides the prohibition of *yichud*. Therefore, it should be forbidden for the extra person to desecrate the Shabbos to go along if the only reason is to avoid *yichud*.

Because of this question, the Shem Aryeh seeks to strike a balance. He writes that if the prohibition in question is only rabbinic, then it may be desecrated to avoid *yichud*. However, it would not be permitted to do a Torah prohibition to avoid an issue of *yichud*. A contemporary of the Shem Aryeh, Rabbi Shlomo Kluger, agreed with this approach.[21]

Based on this approach, we need to determine whether an additional passenger in a car on Shabbos violates a Torah or rabbinic prohibition.[22]

Techum Shabbos

One of the issues with travel on Shabbos is leaving the *techum*. The Torah writes that "a person should not leave his place on Shabbos."[23] It is learned from here that it is prohibited to travel from one's place of dwelling on Shabbos. The halachah is that it is prohibited to travel 2,000 *amos* (approx. 3,500 feet) from the city limits on Shabbos. Although the law derives from a verse in the Torah, there is nonetheless a disagreement whether it has the status of being considered a Torah prohibition or not. Even according to the opinions that it is, the 2,000 *amos* measurement is definitely rabbinic. The Torah prohibition would only be violated when leaving an area of twelve *mil*, which is approximately nine miles.[24]

---

21 *Tuv Taam Vada'as*, cited in *Otzar HaPoskim*.

22 The parameters of when car travel is an issue of *yichud* are beyond the scope of this article. See *Igros Moshe*, Even HaEzer 4:65:3.

23 *Shemos* 16:29; see *Shulchan Aruch*, Orach Chaim 397.

24 Based on the *Igros Moshe's* calculation.

Car Travel on Shabbos

Operating a car entails a Torah prohibition of *ma'avir* — kindling a fire. This is because fuel is added to the engine fire each time the gas pedal is pressed. However, being a passenger doesn't necessarily transgress a prohibition. First of all, it is doubtful if any additional fuel is being used because of the passenger's weight. Secondly, even if the car does burn more gas because of the additional passenger, it is hardly noticeable, and one's action needs to be significant in order to violate a Torah prohibition.[25]

Emotional Support

It is important to point out that our entire discussion relates to when it makes no difference to the patient if someone accompanies him or not. However, more often this is not the case. The patient usually wants someone to accompany him or her for emotional support.[26]

Conclusion

In most situations, accompanying the patient as a passenger to avoid *yichud* only involves rabbinic prohibitions. Therefore, in those situations it is permitted. This is especially true if the patient needs another person to accompany him to calm him, provide medical information, or ensure personal safety.

---

25 See *Chayei Odom*, Meleches Ma'avir (*eino miskavein klal*); *Minchas Shlomo* 1:91:10 regarding Shabbos elevators.

26 This is the concept of *yisuvai daita*; see *Mishnah Berurah* 330:4.

GENERAL SHABBOS QUESTIONS

Shabbos Shift and Lifnei Iver

Q: Is it permitted to request a weekday shift if by doing so it may cause a Jewish person to work on Shabbos?

A: The underlying concept involved in this question is the parameters of *lifnei iver* and *misayeia*, the prohibition to cause or have a supportive role in another person's transgression. We will develop how these concepts apply to such situations.

Lifnei Iver

The Torah writes: "*lifnei iver lo sitain michshol* — you should not cause a person to stumble." The Sages learned from here that it is prohibited to cause another person to transgress one of the mitzvos. However, Tosfos in *Avodah Zarah* explains that the Torah prohibition of *lifnei iver* is only when the prohibition would not be transgressed without your help. However, if your role is only supportive, meaning that the transgression would still happen anyway, it is not a Torah prohibition to give assistance.[27] Nonetheless, the Rosh in *Shabbos* writes that there still is a rabbinic prohibition to have a supportive role,[28] because assisting in such a situation nonetheless contradicts one's obligation to make sure each Jewish person keeps the Torah.

Rabbi Yaakov Etlinger's Discusssion

In 1863, Rabbi Yaakov Etlinger of Altoona, Germany, was asked a question by the Rabbi of Wurzburg. Is it permitted to hire a non-Jewish printer to print a book if he employs Jewish workers who work on Shabbos? Perhaps hiring this printer will cause the Jewish workers to work on Shabbos. Furthermore, the inquirer added, it could at least be an issue of lending aid to a transgression.[29]

First, Rabbi Etlinger addresses the Torah prohibition of *lifnei iver*, causing a transgression. He points out that the printer has plenty of other work for them to do. Therefore, it does not need to be assumed that by hiring the printer the customer is causing additional Shabbos desecration.

In a similar vein, Rabbi Moshe Feinstein discusses if an observant doctor may switch a Saturday shift with a Jewish nonobservant doctor.[30] Superficially, it would seem that this is causing a Jew to desecrate Shabbos and violates *lifnei iver*. However, Rabbi Feinstein points out that even if the doctor is not working he may anyway be doing various prohibited *melachos* — forbidden Shabbos activities, so switching the shift would not really cause any additional desecration of Shabbos. Therefore, causing him to go to work on Shabbos may not be considered *lifnei iver*.

Misayeia — Aiding before the Time of the Transgression

There is an interesting discussion about renting an apartment to a nonobservant Jew. The concern is that the landlord is considered aiding in the tenant's desecration of Shabbos on the premises. As we have

27 6b, s.v. *minayin*.

28 1:1; see also *Shulchan Aruch*, Yoreh Dei'ah 151:6; Shach 6.

29 *Binyan Tzion* 1:15.

30 *Igros Moshe*, Orach Chaim 4:79.

learned, there would not be an issue of *lifnei iver* if there are other apartments available. The remaining issue would be the rabbinic prohibition of *misayeia* — lit. assisting. This prohibits lending aid even if the prohibition is going to happen anyway. However, some understand that the issue of *misayeia* is only if the aid is given at the time of the prohibition. They reason that aid given before the time of the actual transgression is too detached to be an issue. Therefore, since the landlord rents the apartment long before Shabbos, this is not an issue of *misayeia* either.[31]

Rabbi Etlinger used this concept to address the issue of *misayeia* in the case of the printer. He wrote that since the work was given to the printer long before Shabbos, there is no issue of *misayeia*.

Items Not Inherently Connected to a Transgression

There are a number of additional factors that could detract from a situation being considered *lifnei iver* or *misayeia*.

Rabbi Moshe Feinstein understands that the prohibition of *lifnei iver* is possibly only when the item being given is intrinsically linked to a transgression — e.g., giving pork to someone who will eat it. However, an apartment is not inherently connected to Shabbos desecration. If it would be, one could ask how it is permitted to sell a pot to a person who does not keep kosher. The customer will surely use it to transgress the prohibition of cooking milk and meat together. Therefore, based on this approach, Rabbi Feinstein explains that a pot does not necessarily have to cook nonkosher food. Therefore, renting an apartment or selling cookware is not considered an act of *lifnei iver*.[32] Along these lines, the Ksav Sofer writes that a combination of an item not being inherently connected to the prohibition and not being involved at the time of the transgression removes both issues of *lifnei iver* and *misayeia*.[33]

Other Considerations

Rabbi Aharon Kotler and Rabbi Ovadia Yosef both write that the

---

31 *Maharsham* 2:184.

32 *Igros Moshe*, Yoreh Dei'ah 1:72.

33 See *Yesodei Yeshurun*, Hilchos Pesach.

issue of *lifnei iver* is only if it is certain that a prohibition will be transgressed. However, if it is not clear that a transgression will happen, it is not considered *lifnei iver*.[34]

Another important point is that according to the opinion of the Shach, the issue of *misayeia* is only relevant regarding a person who is normally careful about this prohibition.[35] However, this restriction does not apply to aiding a person who is not careful in general about that prohibition. While others disagree with this approach, it is an important opinion.

Rabbi Shlomo Zalman Auerbach and Rabbi Moshe Feinstein point out that the fundamental issue of *misayeia* is in helping someone in wrongdoing. Therefore, if by aiding the person, it will prevent them from transgressing greater prohibitions, it may be viewed as an act of separating a Jew from transgression, not aiding.[36]

Conclusion

Many of these factors may apply to our question and could permit requesting a weekday shift:

- The first consideration is that there are a number of doubts involved. Perhaps a non-Jew will get that slot. Even if a Jewish person is assigned to the Shabbos shift, it is possible that he will trade with someone else.
- Furthermore, as Rabbi Feinstein pointed out, the person may be doing *melachah* anyway if not working. For these reasons it may not be an issue of *lifnei iver*.
- Additionally, the shift may not necessarily entail Shabbos desecration at all. Even if it does, it may be in a form that is permitted, such as in situations of *pikuach nefesh* or those that violate rabbinic prohibitions, which may be permitted in various situations (see footnote).[37]

---

34 See *Shu"t Mishnas Rebbe Aharon* #3; *Yabia Omer* 7:7:2.

35 Yoreh Dei'ah 151:6.

36 *Igros Moshe*, Yoreh Dei'ah 1:72, s.v. *al kol panim*; *Minchas Shlomo* 1:35:1.

37 Rabbi Moshe Sternbuch (*Teshuvos VeHanhagos* 3:357) points out that even for *tzar baalei*

- As far as *misayeia*, there are a number of considerations. According to the Shach, there is no issue of *misayeia* with a non-observant person. Furthermore, requesting the shift is not at the time of prohibition and also may not be directly connected to Shabbos. These factors therefore could mitigate the issues of *misayeia* and possibly *lifnei iver*.

Billing for Services Rendered on Shabbos

Q: Is it permitted to bill a patient or the insurance company for services rendered on Shabbos? What about charging for materials? Does it make a difference if I service them before or after Shabbos as well? Does the weekday service need to be directly related to the service provided on Shabbos?

A: We will explain the concept of *schar Shabbos*, the prohibition of receiving payment for work done on Shabbos, and how it may apply to this setting.

Schar Shabbos

The Sages restricted many forms of business on Shabbos because it may lead to writing and other prohibitions. One of these restrictions is *schar Shabbos*, not to accept payment for work done on Shabbos. However, they limited this rabbinic safeguard to where the payment is solely for work done on Shabbos. Therefore, in our situation, if a single payment covers both the Shabbos and weekday visits, there is no restriction. The leniency of a combined Shabbos and non-Shabbos

chaim — pain to animals, a rabbinic prohibition is sometimes permitted on Shabbos.

payment is called *havla'ah* — lit. swallow. Because the Shabbos payment is "swallowed" with the weekday payment, it is permitted.[38] As such, even if the two visits are unrelated, as long as the payment is not solely for the care given on Shabbos, it would seem that it may be accepted. Furthermore, it is only prohibited to profit from services rendered on Shabbos, but there is no obligation to incur a loss. For this reason, it is always permitted to bill for the cost of supplies.[39]

The Chazzan's Wages

There is a lot of rabbinic discussion regarding the wages of a professional chazzan (cantor). Is the chazzan permitted to accept payment from the synagogue for his services, since they are only rendered on Shabbos? The *Shulchan Aruch* cites an opinion that accepting payment was never prohibited for a mitzvah.[40] However, some opinions do not agree with this dispensation.

The *Mishnah Berurah* writes that a midwife may charge for her services on Shabbos.[41] Firstly, providing medical care is a mitzvah and according to many opinions it is permitted to accept payment for a mitzvah-related service. Although this is not universally accepted, there is a second reason to permit the midwife to accept payment. There is a concern that the midwife may become lax in providing care because subconsciously she knows that that she will not be paid for services rendered on Shabbos. As such, the rabbis lifted the prohibition for a midwife to accept Shabbos wages.

Contemporary Sources

The Har Tzvi and *Teshuvos VeHanhagos* apply the leniency of a midwife to doctors and other medical care providers. However, they caution that depending on the situation, there may not be a real concern that the care provider will come to be lax in the future. Therefore, it is best to use the accepted leniency of *havla'ah*, which avoids the problem entirely.[42]

---

38 See *Shulchan Aruch*, Orach Chaim 306:5 for general concepts.

39 See also *Nodah BeYehudah* 2, Orach Chaim 26 about charging for supplies.

40 *Shulchan Aruch* loc.cit. 306:4–5.

41 *Mishnah Berurah* 306:24.

42 *Har Tzvi*, Orach Chaim 1:204; *Teshuvos VeHanhagos* 2:194.

Injections on Shabbos

Q: Is it permitted to give an injection on Shabbos in a non-life-threatening situation?

A: The main concern with giving an injection on Shabbos is that the puncture may cause the patient to bleed, which might violate the *melachah* of *shechitah*.

Let us review some basic concepts:[43]

- All the forbidden forms of work on Shabbos are derived from the thirty-nine forms of craftsmanship used to build the Mishkan (Tabernacle). In order to be liable for transgressing one of these forbidden forms of work on Shabbos, it must be done intentionally. If it was not done intentionally, it is called *davar she'eino miskavein*. According to many opinions, *davar she'eino miskavein* is only permitted if it is not certain that the *melachah* will result from this action. If it is certain, this is called *psik raisha*, which is a rabbinic prohibition if the outcome is not wanted (*lo ni'cha lei*), but could be a Torah prohibition if the outcome is wanted (*ni'cha lei*).
- For a *melachah* done on Shabbos to be considered having violated a Torah prohibition, it must be done for the same purpose as the act was done in the Mishkan (Tabernacle). This concept is called *melachah she'eino tzrichah legufo*. If not, the act nonetheless violates a rabbinic prohibition. In the Mishkan, juice or blood was extracted purposely to be used in different dyes. Therefore, if there was no intention to draw out the liquid or to use it, it would not be a Torah prohibition.

Let us apply these principles to our case:

---

43 See *Mishnah Berurah* 320:18.

- If the intent is not to draw blood at all, and it is not for sure that the puncture will cause bleeding, it is permitted. This is the concept of *davar she'eino miskavein*.
- If the puncture will definitely cause bleeding, according to many opinions this is considered a *psik raisha* and is a rabbinic prohibition. Therefore, it should be avoided.
- Rabbi Yitzchok Elchonon Specktor maintains that a *psik raisha* could be permitted for a rabbinic prohibition when the outcome is not wanted (*lo ni'cha lei*).[44] According to this approach, it could be permitted to give an injection even if it will definitely bleed. As we learned, giving an injection would only be a rabbinic prohibition because there is no intention to use the blood. As such, even if it will certainly bleed, but is unintentional, it is permitted.

Rapid Throat Cultures on Shabbos

Q: Is it permitted to give a rapid throat culture on Shabbos?

A: There are two interesting parts to this question:

- Does creating the solution and causing the test strips to change colors involve one of the thirty-nine *melachos* of Shabbos?
- Is testing and treating strep throat considered *pikuach nefesh*? If strep throat is left untreated, it can be very dangerous. However, many people may routinely wait a day before seeking medical attention.

44 *Be'er Yitzchok*, Orach Chaim #15.

Is This Tzoveia?

Causing the test strips to change color could possibly violate the prohibition of *tzoveia* — dying. However, there are a number of reasons why these types of tests are not so similar to the way dying was done in the Mishkan. This discussion also applies to urine test strips.

In the Mishkan, the wool and linen were dyed with blue, red, and purple for both the coverings and the clothing of the High Priest. It is important to point out that the intention was to permanently beautify the fabric with these dyes. For this reason a white cloth napkin that becomes stained with grape juice, for example, is not a Torah prohibition as there is no intention to beatify the fabric with the stain. This concept is called *tzviah derech lichluch* — coloring by soiling the garment. Because this type of coloring is the exact opposite of a purposeful *melachah*, many opinions completely permit it. Even according to the stringent view, if the surface being soiled is disposable, like paper napkins, it is permitted. This is because it is clear that there is no intent to dye the material.[45] Returning to our question, could disposable test strips be compared to paper napkins?

The test strips raise an interesting question. When napkins become soiled, they are not being colored for any purpose. On the other hand, the color of the test strips provides important information. We definitely want the color to appear to let us know if the test is positive or negative. However, the coloring does not serve to enhance the strip itself, but instead serves a different reason altogether. Furthermore, the strip will be disposed of immediately after the dying.

Another point to consider is that some view the coloring process as being an indirect result. This is because the color is not applied to the strip but appears on its own due to a chemical reaction. It also does not happen immediately.

As with many of these types of questions, the arguments are convincing enough to assert that such tests are not a Torah prohibition.

---

45 See *Mishnah Berurah* 320:58–59.

However, it may be a rabbinic prohibition. Therefore, one should only be lenient if there is a real need to do the test on Shabbos.[46]

Makeh Bipatish?

A friend raised the issue whether mixing the two types of drops to create the solution for the test is considered *makeh bipatish*, the *melachah* of a craftsman putting the finishing touch on an item. Is creating a solution significant enough to be considered *makeh bipatish*? It does not seem so. This question is reminiscent of the discussions about carbonating water to make seltzer on Shabbos that can be found in halachic discussions beginning in the late 1800s. The Minchas Yitzchak rules leniently because the actual water is not being changed but is just infused with a gas.[47] He contends that if one forgot to do so before Shabbos it may be done on Shabbos. In our case, mixing the drops is far better because there is no noticeable change at the point of combining the two drops. As such, it should not be an issue.

Curable Infections — Is Strep Throat Pikuach Nefesh?

We will begin this part of our discussion with considering if a dangerous infection that is easily curable with antibiotics, like strep throat, is considered *pikuach nefesh*. There is a strong argument that from a halachic standpoint, the availability of antibiotics does not diminish the seriousness of the situation. The Rashba writes that *birchas hagomel* — the blessing made after recovering from a dangerous illness — is made even after recovering from an ailment that it is common to recover from. This is still considered a dangerous situation because the person's life was still in danger.[48] Similarly, Rabbi Moshe Feinstein writes that *birchas hagomel* is said even after domestic flights.[49] He considered all air travel to be inherently dangerous. The fact that the vast majority of flights land safely does not eliminate the danger.

---

46 See *Shemiras Shabbos K'hilchasah* 33:20; *Shearim Mitzuyanim BeHalachah* 91:7; *Be'er Moshe* 8:24.

47 9:33.

48 Cited in *Mishnah Berurah* 219:26.

49 *Igros Moshe*, Orach Chaim 2:14.

While it is not common practice to follow this position, we can learn from here that the availability of a cure doesn't take away from an ailment being considered dangerous. On the other hand, the Talmud in *Sanhedrin* writes that a person is not guilty of murder for inflicting a wound that there is medicine available to heal.[50] Apparently the availability of medical attention diminishes the perpetrator's act from murder to assault. This would indicate the opposite — that the availability of antibiotics detracts from an ailment being considered *pikuach nefesh*.[51]

Rabbi Auerbach's Approach

Rabbi Shlomo Zalman Auerbach in *Minchas Shlomo* raises another point.[52] Some people overreact and run to the hospital for the most minor ailment. Others wait until it seems more severe. Being that this is so subjective, how do we determine when something is considered *pikuach nefesh*? He tries to strike a balance and writes that the litmus test is how careful people are during the week to treat this particular ailment. If during the week it is normally taken care of right away, it could be done on Shabbos. However, if during the week this person would wait to take care of it, then they should not desecrate Shabbos to do so.

Superficially, Rabbi Auerbach's reasoning seems arbitrary. The definition of *pikuach nefesh* remains subjective and whimsical. However, a deeper understanding of the concept of *pikuach nefesh* provides greater appreciation for this definition.

The source of *pikuach nefesh* is from the verse "*ve'chai ba'hem* — you shall **live** [with the Torah]." The Rambam explains that the rules of the Torah are "merciful and kind" and should not cause a loss of human life in any way.[53] It should follow that this dispensation allows for human error and opinion. Taking this point further, the objective of the Torah is not to be a medical guide. Therefore, it gives people the room needed so that protecting and preserving life does not conflict with their Torah

---

50 77b.

51 For more discussion about this concept, see *Divrei Malkiel* 3:26, which deals with fasting on Tishah B'Av during a cholera epidemic.

52 2:37.

53 *Shabbos* 2:3.

obligations. As such, people's normal behavior during the week (when Shabbos is not a factor) is a good barometer, albeit imperfect, to gauge what is really necessary. This judgment will inherently vary from person to person and situation to situation, but nonetheless this is exactly what the Torah permitted.

Conclusion

The rapid strep test does not pose a serious halachic issue. Therefore, if there is any reason for urgency, especially with children, the elderly, or a risk of spreading infection to others, one should not hesitate to do what is necessary. However, if the test is being done out of mere convenience, it should be avoided.

X-Rays and Digital Imaging on Shabbos

Q: Is the exposure of film to X-rays on Shabbos considered an act of "writing"? What about developing film? How does halachah view digital imaging?

A: Any usage of electrical machinery on Shabbos can involve a myriad of potential problems. This discussion focuses on if photography is considered writing.

Early Discussions about Photography

By the late 1800s, halachic questions about photography started appearing in rabbinic works. For example, can a photograph be used to identify a body to permit the wife to remarry? One of the first discussions about photography on Shabbos is by Rabbi Elazar Dovid

Greenwald (d. 1928) of Hungary, in *Keren LeDovid*.[54] It was addressed to his student Chaim Weider and discusses taking a passport photograph on Shabbos. Chaim would be required to bring a photograph if he was called to report to the Hungarian army on Shabbos.

Rabbi Greenwald first addresses if the exposure of film to light is considered an act of writing. One could argue that since the photographer doesn't actively create the image but rather lets in the light, it is not an act of writing. However, he concludes that since the image is an immediate result of the person's action, it is still considered an act of writing. Therefore, the act of taking the photograph is forbidden. He then addresses if it is permitted to have a non-Jew take the picture. Is it permitted to stand in front of the camera and allow oneself to be photographed? He concludes that in such extenuating circumstances, it is permitted.[55]

Rabbi Moshe Feinstein on the other hand considers photography an act of writing on Shabbos.[56] He explains that the laws of Shabbos are different than the laws of writing a Torah scroll. On Shabbos the prohibition is to cause the creation of an image, therefore a photograph is considered writing. However, for a Torah scroll to be valid it must be written in the traditional and literal sense. Therefore a photographic image is not valid for a Torah scroll. Rabbi Gedalia Felder of Toronto, in *Yesodei Yeshurun*, also reaches the same conclusion.

Developing Film

Contemporary sources raise an important point. Photography is only considered an act of writing when the image is created directly by the exposure to light without any other process. The old Polaroid cameras used to work that way. However, often the image only becomes visible through the chemical process of developing the film. As such, the direct outcome of taking the picture is not visible and cannot be considered an act of writing. This raises a new question. Is developing film an act of writing?

---

54 #102.

55 Rabbi Yonosan Shteif, cited in *Shearim Mitzuyanim BeHalachah* concurs with this point.

56 Orach Chaim 4:40:10.

The Pri Megadim deals with a similar question.[57] People would send secret messages by writing with uncooked milk on a piece of paper. The milk cannot be seen but when the paper is placed near a fire the letters reappear. He questions if there is a prohibition to make the letters reappear. He contends it is only a rabbinic prohibition because it is not a regular act of writing.

It would seem, based on this approach, that developing film is a rabbinic prohibition, not a Torah offense. However, though *Shevet HaLevi* contends that developing film is not writing, he argues that it would be *makeh bipatish*.[58]

Phonographs, Records, and Tapes

In order to formulate an approach to digital imaging, we will first review some of the discussions about recording on a phonograph, record, or tape. In the late 1800s, Rabbi Shmuel Shmelkish of Lemberg in *Beis Yitzchak* was one of the first rabbis to address the use of electricity and recording devices (phonograph) on Shabbos. He writes that recording on Shabbos is like making an imprint into wax or clay, and as such is included in the *melachah* of writing.

Rabbi Yaakov Breisch of Zurich, in *Chelkas Yaakov*,[59] took this approach very literally and prohibited discarding any records and tapes that have the name of Hashem recorded on them. Rabbi Breisch equated the indiscernible imprint on these items to a written name of Hashem. He wrote: "what is the difference between the sense of hearing or the sense of seeing?" Meaning that it makes no difference that the imprint cannot be seen since it can be played and heard. He compared erasing a tape recording to a holy book written in braille for the seeing impaired. Just as G-d's name cannot be erased in other languages, it cannot be erased in braille because the imprint is meaningful. Similarly,

---

57 In *Mishbitzos Zahav* 340:2.

58 The Pri Megadim omits discussing whether writing the original message is a Torah or rabbinic prohibition. This seems to indicate that in his opinion it is neither. The Avnei Nezer also demonstrates that causing an invisible imprint to become visible is not a new act of writing and would not be a Torah prohibition if done on Shabbos.

59 3:98.

if the imprint is on a tape or record, that imprint is also meaningful and cannot be erased.

Other contemporary halachic sources do not view a recording as a name of G-d.[60] Rabbi Moshe Feinstein writes in *Igros Moshe* that since there are no noticeable letters, it does not need *genizah* — burial, but nonetheless should be discarded in a respectful manner.[61] Similarly, the *Piskei Teshuvah* (printed in Poland) discusses if a holy book on microfilm has *kedushah*. He writes that because the image cannot be seen by the naked eye, it is not considered as having letters. Therefore it does not have the status of a holy book.

According to this more lenient approach, it seems that there is an important difference between Hashem's name written in Braille or on a record or tape. A recording, unlike braille, is not in a printed form discernible by human beings. This is similar to microfilm that cannot be viewed without the aid of a machine. As such, it is not considered a form of expression bearing the prohibition of erasing G-d's name. In the same vein, the Arugas HaBosem writes that recording on a phonograph on Shabbos is not a Torah prohibition but a rabbinic one. This view would be more in line with these sources.

Digital Imaging

Based on the above discussion, we can now consider digital imaging on Shabbos. According to many *poskim*, an imprint that is not discernible to the naked eye is not significant. Therefore, creating a digital image should not be considered an act of writing. As such, digital imaging is probably not a Torah prohibition, but a rabbinic one.

Conclusion

Creating a digital image or taking an X-Ray without developing it would be a rabbinic prohibition. While the difference is more theoretical, the Minchas Yitzchak used this approach when dealing with a doctor who may have to take X-rays in situations that are not clearly

---

60 See *Yabia Omer* 4, Yoreh Dei'ah 20 for an extensive discussion.

61 *Igros Moshe*, Yoreh Dei'ah 1:173, Orach Chaim 3:31.

pikuach nefesh. He writes that if it is only a rabbinic prohibition, it is more lenient. Nonetheless, with today's sophisticated machinery, it is doubtful whether there are no Torah prohibitions involved in operating them on Shabbos.

Another point to consider: it does not seem that a patient transgresses a Torah prohibition by allowing himself to be X-rayed by a non-Jewish technician. This may be helpful when dealing with situations that do not clearly fall into the category of *pikuach nefesh*.

Stitches on Shabbos and the Melachah of Tofair (Sewing)

Q: Does stitching a wound on Shabbos violate one of the thirty-nine *melachos*?

A: This discussion focuses on whether stitching a wound on Shabbos involves a Torah or a rabbinic prohibition.

Introduction

This discussion is more theoretical than previous cases of medical protocol. On the one hand, in a situation of *pikuach nefesh*, medical care is permitted regardless of the severity of the prohibition. On the flip side, when it is not urgent, then even a rabbinic prohibition may not be violated.

However, this particular question is important because whether stitching a wound is a Torah or rabbinic issue makes a difference in the halachic decision-making process. For example, *poskim* use a lower threshold of risk when permitting a *melachah* that is only a rabbinic prohibition. Additionally, we have discussed that nonessential care that is only a rabbinic prohibition may be permitted for a seriously ill patient. Furthermore, in situations of *kavod habrios* — human dignity, it may be permitted to violate a rabbinic prohibition but not a Torah transgression. This could apply to stitches where there could be bad scarring if the wound is not stitched properly.

Here are some important sources:

Rabbi Yechezkel Abramsky's Position

Rabbi Yechezkel Abramsky was a famous *talmid* of Rabbi Chaim Brisker and head of the London Beis Din. He reportedly said that there is no Torah prohibition in stitching human skin. His reasoning was because such forms of sewing were not found in the Mishkan.[62]

Machlokes Rishonim?

It is possible that whether or not the *melachah* of sewing applies to skin is a dispute between the Rishonim. The Talmud considers a specific procedure of draining a wound, called *mapis mursa*, a Torah prohibition. According to Rashi, it is considered the *melachah* of building. However, the Rambam gives a different explanation. He writes that it is the *melachah* of *makeh bipatish* — a craftsman finishing his craft. The Avnei Nezer understands that their dispute is whether there is a concept of building on the human body. Rashi maintains that a procedure done to the body can still be considered building, while the Rambam feels that this is too removed from how building was done in the Mishkan. Therefore, he considers it to be a different *melachah* of *makeh bipatish*.[63] It is possible that this discussion extends to the *melachah* of sewing as well. Sewing is normally done with fabric. Is human skin too different? Rabbi Abramsky maintained that it is. As we will see, Rabbi Shlomo Zalman Auerbach felt differently.

Rabbi Shlomo Zalman Auerbach's Approach

Rabbi Shlomo Zalman Auerbach in *Minchas Shlomo* raises the possibility that the prohibition of *tofair*, applies even to items that are

---

62 Cited in *Nishmas Avraham*, Orach Chaim 340; and *Tzitz Eliezer* 20:18.

63 Interestingly, the *Shulchan Aruch* quotes the Rambam, not Rashi.

not normally sewn.[64] He based this on the fact that gluing items like leather, paper, and wood are included in this *melachah*.[65] As such, it could apply to human skin as well. He also points out that writing on human skin violates the *melachah* of *koseiv* — writing. However, he acknowledges that his approach is not conclusive, as we find that applying a dye to human skin is only a rabbinic prohibition of *tzoveia* — dyeing. Nonetheless, he concludes that stitching human skin is possibly a Torah prohibition.

Is This a Sofek?

The approach of the *Minchas Shlomo* does not explain the numerous contradictions whether various *melachos* apply to the human body or not. For this reason, the Shevet HaLevi,[66] Chut Shani, and Rabbi Yosef Shalom Elyashiv,[67] consider it to be a *sofek* — a halachic doubt — if *tofair* applies to human skin (*sofek d'Oraisa*). However, Rabbi Yisroel Yaakov Fisher in *Even Yisrael* comments that we do not find the prohibition of *tofair* on living creatures or human beings.[68] He writes that it is probable that there is no Torah prohibition of *tofair* on human skin. It is interesting that Rabbi Fisher is not deterred by the fact that items like leather, wood, and paper have this prohibition.[69]

Must We Assume This to Be a Melachah?

There may be a difference of approach between Rabbi Auerbach and Rabbi Fisher. How do we view forms of craftsmanship not clearly found in the Mishkan? Are they assumed to be a Torah prohibition unless there is a decisive proof otherwise? Or, the opposite, the very fact that we don't find such forms of the *melachah* allows us to assume that

---

64 2:35.

65 See Biur Halachah 340.

66 9:74:2.

67 Cited in *Nishmas Avraham*.

68 8:27.

69 In general, the *Minchas Shlomo's* assumption that these items are not normally sewn may be questionable. Leather definitely is sewn, and paper could very well have been normally sewn just like today large paper sacks are sewn. Wood in the form of reeds was commonly woven together in a form of sewing, as mentioned in the Biur Halachah.

they are not Torah prohibitions unless proven so? Rabbi Auerbach is apparently taking the view that although it is unclear if stitching skin is included in *tofair*, we are nonetheless compelled to assume so. On the other hand, Rabbi Fisher is assuming, based on the lack of evidence, that it is not included in *tofair*.[70]

Rabbi Waldenberg's Approach

Rabbi Eliezer Waldenberg in *Tzitz Eliezer* supports the position of Rabbi Yechezkel Abramsky that sewing human skin is not a Torah prohibition.[71] He seeks to reconcile why writing on skin is a *melachah* whereas coloring and dyeing skin is not.[72] He points out that when writing on skin, the main focus is on the words and the skin is just the surface. Therefore, even though writing on live skin is not the norm, the essence of the *melachah*, the words, is not that different. Therefore it is still considered a Torah prohibition. However, when dyeing, the surface being colored is central to the *melachah*. The focus of the *melachah* is to beautify this surface. As such, the fact that it is unusual to dye live skin is much more significant. For this reason, it is not a Torah prohibition. Rabbi Issur Zalman Meltzer, in *Even HaAzel*, uses a similar approach to explain why some forms of building are a Torah prohibition while others are not.[73]

The *Tzitz Eliezer* applies this reasoning to sewing skin. Unlike the *melachah* of writing, *tofair* is all about repairing the surface. Therefore, our case of sewing skin should not be included in the Torah prohibition of *tofair*.

A Different Objective

Rabbi Moshe Sternbuch in *Teshuvos VeHanhagos* makes an important argument why stitching human skin should not be a Torah prohibition.[74]

---

70 On this general question, note that in *Igros Moshe* (Orach Chaim 1:122:6), Rabbi Moshe Feinstein assumes there is no *melachah* of building with fabric and material simply because "we don't find a concept of building with clothing since material does not stand on its own."

71 20:18.

72 Rabbi Waldenberg also points out that the Torah prohibition of tattoos demonstrates that writing on human skin was an accepted societal norm. Dyeing human skin may have been different.

73 *Shabbos* 10:17.

74 3:103.

In truth, the objective of stitching a wound is very different than a tailor stitching a suit. With regular sewing, the purpose of the stitches is to permanently hold the two sides of the garment together. When stitching human skin, the objective is not to forever fix the body with stitches. On the contrary, we do not want the stitches to remain forever. The objective is just to facilitate the human body's natural healing process. For this reason it should not be considered the Torah prohibition of sewing.[75]

Makeh Bipatish

Rabbi Shmuel Wosner in *Shevet HaLevi* raised the issue of whether stitching a wound is considered *makeh bipatish*. This is an interesting point because the Rambam considered a drainage procedure for wounds to be *makeh bipatish*. We see that *makeh bipatish* definitely applies to the human body. However, there are two reasons why stitching a wound may be different.

- There is much discussion about the level of completion required to classify an act as *makeh bipatish*.[76] However, it would seem that to be considered *makeh bipatish*, there must be a meaningful creation at some level, e.g., creating drainage passage in a wound. However, stitches do not seem to be a creation. It is just a way of bringing two sides together. Unlike a drainage system, stitches have no intrinsic function. As such, it is difficult to compare it to *makeh bipatish* where the craftsman completes an object.
- According to many Acharonim, a *melachah* that could fall into two of the thirty-nine categories can not classify as both. Rather we judge it based on the one it is most similar to. Draining a wound is not comparable to anything other than *makeh bipatish*. However, stitching a wound is most similar to regular stitching than to anything else. As such it could only be considered *tofair*, not *makeh bipatish*, and thus all the previous discussions apply.[77]

---

75 In consultation with Rabbi Dovid Feinstein, he found this argument to be quite convincing.

76 See *Igros Moshe*, Orach Chaim 1:122; *Bircas Avraham* on *Shabbos* 75a, 122b; *Even HaAzel* on *Shabbos* 10:17.

77 See *Tzitz Eliezer* loc. cit. for discussion.

Conclusion

There are various differences between stitching a wound and the stitching done in the Mishkan. Therefore contemporary halachic sources cannot definitively consider it to be a Torah prohibition of *tofair*. However, it is most definitely a rabbinic prohibition. Furthermore, stitching a wound on Shabbos involves other questions of tying knots, cutting thread and trimming skin, which will be discussed in the coming pages.

Additional Questions about Stitching a Wound on Shabbos

Q: a. Is tying knots in the process of stitching a wound a Torah prohibition of koshair — knotting?

b. Does revision, i.e., trimming the edges of the wound, violate the *melachah* of *gozeiz* — shearing?

A: We will continue to examine when a procedure is a Torah or rabbinic prohibition.

When Is Tying a Knot a Torah Prohibition?

In creating the Mishkan, the trappers of the chilazon fish made nets with knots. From here it is learned that tying an expert knot is forbidden on Shabbos. The Torah prohibition of knotting therefore has two criteria: it must be an expert knot and long-lasting. The Rishonim seek to define how permanent the knot must be to be prohibited. They give different amounts of time. However, their entire discussion is when the knot is temporary enough to be permitted. All agree that only a knot that is meant to be left indefinitely transgress a Torah prohibition.[78]

Stitching a Wound

With this in mind, we can consider our question about stitches. Stitches either are removed after a number of days or eventually dissolve. As such, these knots are not permanent and seemingly do not violate a Torah prohibition.

However, the question has been raised that although the stitches are removed and discarded, the actual knot remains tied. As such, is this considered a permanent knot? Rabbi Shlomo Zalman Auerbach and Rabbi Moshe Sternbuch dismiss this concern. They understand that the function of the knot is holding the two ends of the string together. Therefore, if the bind is severed, the knot is functionless and is not considered permanent anymore.[79]

Disposable Items

There is an additional reason not to consider the knot that is thrown out a Torah prohibition, even though it is never untied. The Maharil Diskin wonders if a knot can only be considered permanent if the intent is to *use* the knot indefinitely.[80] However, if it is discarded and no one cares if it exists anymore, it would not be considered making a permanent knot.[81]

The Tzitz Eliezer builds on this idea. He contends that assembling disposable syringes and IV tubing on Shabbos is not considered a permanent act of building even though they will not be taken apart. The fact that they are thrown away declassifies it from being a *melachah*.[82]

---

78 See *Tur* and *Aruch HaShulchan*, Orach Chaim #317.

79 *Minchas Shlomo* 2:35; *Teshuvos VeHanhagos* 3:103.

80 Cited in *Tzitz Eliezer* 16:7.

81 He brings a possible indication of this concept from the red string tied to the horns of the *sa'ir le'azazel* — the goat thrown to Azazel in the Yom Kippur service in the Beis HaMikdosh. The Maharil Diskin wonders how they could tie the string to the horns on Yom Kippur as it violates the *melachah* of knotting. He writes that perhaps because it is being discarded it is not considered permanent and does not violate a Torah prohibition.

82 Rabbi Waldenberg also discusses this with regards to disposable diapers that have adhesives

Based on this approach, the very fact that the knotted stitches are thrown out reduces its severity from being a Torah prohibition.[83]

Revision — Trimming the Edges of the Wound

We will now consider if trimming the edges of the wound violates the *melachah* of *gozeiz* — shearing. According to most Rishonim, a *melachah* done for a different purpose than the one done in the Mishkan is not a Torah prohibition. This concept is called *melachah she'eino tzrichah legufah*. Therefore, we need to understand why shearing was done in the process of building the Mishkan. Was it to beautify the hides or to use the wool?

According to Tosfos, the shearing in the Mishkan was in order to use the wool, not to beautify the hides. It follows that cutting fingernails or giving a haircut is not a Torah prohibition. This is because unlike in the Mishkan, there is no intention to use the shorn hair or loose/cut fingernails. However, the Rivosh understands that shearing was also done to prepare the hides for use. As such, if the person is beautified by trimming his hair or fingernails, the act would still be similar to the cutting done in the Mishkan. Therefore, according to the Rivosh, cutting hair or fingernails would be a Torah prohibition.

The *poskim* bring up this dispute between Tosfos and the Rivosh regarding a woman who is going to the mikvah on Friday night and forgot to cut a fingernail. The Magen Avraham follows the lenient opinion of Tosfos. He writes that a non-Jew may cut it for her because cutting fingernails is only a rabbinic transgression. This is based on the concept of *shvus deshvus bemakom mitzvah* (see footnote).[84]

Other *poskim* are concerned that the opinion of the *Shulchan Aruch* and others seems to be stringent like the Rivosh. However, the Biur

---

and other such situations.

83 *Tzitz Eliezer* 15:17, 16:6–7.

84 *Shvus deshvus bemakom mitzvah* means that an action that is only a rabbinic transgression for two reasons is permitted for a mitzvah. According to the Magen Avraham, this rule applies to our situation. A non-Jew doing *melachah* for a Jew on Shabbos is only a rabbinic prohibition, and cutting fingernails is only rabbinic since they will not be used (like Tosfos, not the Rivosh).

Halachah argues that even the Rivosh will agree. In this case, the nails are not being cut to beautify the body. It is being done for a halachic reason, i.e., to remove a possible *chatzitzah* — a separation between the body and the mikvah water.[85] Cutting nails to avoid a *chatzitzah* is not like the cutting that was done in the Mishkan, where the hairs were removed to beautify the hides.

In our case, when the skin is trimmed for wound closure, there is no intention of using the skin. Therefore according to Tosfos this is not a Torah prohibition. Furthermore, even according to the Rivosh, cutting skin to aid in wound closure is very different from getting a manicure! It is possible that even the Rivosh would agree that revision is not a Torah prohibition.

The Melachah of Mechatech — Cutting

Another issue is if cutting the threads while stitching violates the *melachah* of *mechatech* — cutting an item to size. The Rambam writes that the *melachah* of *mechatech* is only a Torah prohibition when done to a specific length. Therefore, cutting *derech hefesk* — just to sever a loose end, is not a Torah prohibition.[86]

When stitching, the doctor may cut the thread in between stitches. If he is not particular on a specific length, it is not a Torah prohibition.

A Final Thought

Rabbi Moshe Feinstein discusses the possible *melachos* involved in using a hearing aid on Shabbos.[87] He then writes: "It is not clear what category of *melachah* it falls into. Therefore we cannot prohibit its use for the elderly and infirmed since there is no definitive prohibition."

This idea may apply to our question as well. Generally we are stringent with the laws of Shabbos. However, in extenuating circumstances, it is difficult to definitively consider stitching a wound as a Torah prohibition because of the lack of clarity on the subject.

---

85 See *Mishnah Berurah* 340 and Biur Halachah there for full discussion.

86 Cited in *Chayei Adam* 36:1.

87 Orach Chaim 4:85.

Kiddush for Person with Health Problems and Celiac Disease

Q: A person has great difficulty drinking wine or grape juice. In addition, the person has celiac disease and cannot have any grain products. What are the options to fulfill the obligation of Kiddush on Shabbos, both Friday night and Shabbos day? How can he fulfill the requirement of *Kiddush bemakom seudah* — having Kiddush in the place of the meal, if he cannot have any bread or *mezonos*?

A: Here are some thoughts on this tricky question:

The Obligation of Kiddush

The Torah instructs us *zachor es yom haShabbos lekadsho* — remember the day of Shabbos to sanctify it. The Torah obligation to recite Kiddush Friday night is derived from this verse. To fulfill this, it is sufficient to simply recite the verses of Kiddush. However, the Sages instituted an obligation to recite them over a cup of wine.[88] They also required it to be recited at a meal of bread or *mezonos*, called *Kiddush bemakom seudah*. The Sages also obligated the recital of Kiddush on Shabbos day as well.

Friday Night Kiddush

As we mentioned, Kiddush should be recited over a cup of wine or grape juice. However, if there is no wine available, the *Shulchan Aruch* writes that Kiddush may be recited over bread.[89] In the event that bread is not available, it is questionable if other beverages may be used. Nonetheless, there is still a mitzvah to recite the verses of Kiddush. However, the full text of Friday night Kiddush should not be said. This is because it includes a brachah on the Shabbos that may be in vain if re-

88 See *Mishnah Berurah* 271:2.

89 *Orach Chaim* 272:9.

cited without wine or bread. Therefore, in our situation, the best option would be for the person to listen to another person recite Kiddush over wine. However, if no one else is available, the Torah obligation of Kiddush should be fulfilled by either praying the *Maariv Shemoneh Esrei* (which includes the verses of *vayichulu hashamayim...*), or at least by reading the relevant verses but omitting the final brachah. Once he has done so, he may eat his other foods.

Shabbos Day Kiddush

We have learned that the Sages instituted the recital of Kiddush over wine on Shabbos day. If no wine is available for Kiddush on Shabbos day, it can be made on beverages classified as *chamar medinah*, an important beverage.[90] Beer and whisky are classic examples of such important beverages, but according to the *Aruch HaShulchan* and *Igros Moshe*, coffee and tea can also qualify. Some consider juice and milk to be *chamar medinah* as well.

The text of the Shabbos day Kiddush does not contain a special brachah — just a few verses and the blessing of the beverage. Therefore, although there are varying opinions on this subject, there is no concern of saying a brachah in vain.

Kiddush Bemakom Seudah

In this situation, the tricky issue is the requirement of having the Kiddush as part of a meal — *Kiddush bemakom seudah*. Generally, to be considered a "meal," it must be bread or a *mezonos* food from the five grains. The *Shulchan Aruch* cites the opinion of the Geonim that drinking an extra glass of wine or grape juice can also be considered a "meal" for this purpose.[91] This would generally work for people with celiac disease who can not have grain but can have grape juice. In our situation, though, the individual can not tolerate either. The *Mishnah Berurah* cites the opinion of the Shiltei Geborim that other foods, like

---

90 *Shulchan Aruch*, Orach Chaim 272:9.

91 Orach Chaim 273:5.

fruit, can also be considered a meal.[92] However, this is a minority opinion and is generally not relied upon. Nonetheless, the *Mishnah Berurah* cites some opinions who rely on the Shiltei Geborim for an ill person for Shabbos day Kiddush only.

Rabbi Moshe Sternbuch in *Teshuvos VeHanhagos* argues that non-*mezonos* foods for a person who cannot have bread or wine due to health issues are considered more important.[93] Therefore, in such situations, more authorities may concur with the view of the Shiltei Geborim to use other staple foods as a "meal."[94]

Stethoscope on Shabbos

Q: Is it permitted to use a stethoscope on Shabbos in a non-*pikuach-nefesh* situation for medical diagnostic purposes? What about non-medical purposes?

A: Here are some pertinent points:

Telescope

Around seven hundred years ago, the Rashba was asked if a telescope could be used on Shabbos.[95] He responded that it is permitted to use it on Shabbos just as it is permitted to read a book of secular knowledge

92 *Mishnah Berurah* 273:26.

93 2:160.

94 This argument is similar to the rationale given for the custom in Chassidic circles to use just a shot glass of whisky for Kiddush. Normally, Kiddush requires a *riviis*, which is about three fluid ounces, not a shot glass that contains only around one fluid ounce. The Taz explains that since whisky is very strong, people consider this to be a significant amount. Therefore, a shot glass is sufficient. Likewise, we could argue that for individuals in our situation, non-*mezonos* foods are more significant and may fulfill the requirement of *Kiddush bemakom seudah*.

95 *Shu"t HaRashba* 1:772.

on Shabbos. Therefore, it does not pose a problem of *muktzah* either. The Rashba adds that we are not concerned that a person would fix it on Shabbos if it breaks.

Rabbi Yosef Karo understands the ruling of the Rashba to possibly be contingent on whether it is even permitted to study subjects other than Torah on Shabbos.[96] The Rambam and Ran are of the opinion that only Torah should be studied on Shabbos. It should follow that a telescope, which is used in pursuing secular knowledge, is forbidden to be used on Shabbos. However, the Rashba, who permitted the telescope, is following his opinion and that of many other Rishonim who permit studying all forms of knowledge on Shabbos. Therefore, it is permitted to pursue this knowledge by using a telescope on Shabbos.

The *Mishnah Berurah* writes that the custom is to follow the lenient opinion.[97] Additionally, the *Mishnah Berurah* cites the opinion of the Vilna Gaon that even according to the Rambam a telescope is not *muktzah*.[98] Based on this discussion it would seem that a stethoscope, which is used to study the heart, is permissible to be used on Shabbos and is not *muktzah*. However, unlike a telescope, it is possibly a measuring device. We will consider this aspect of the question.

Measuring Time

The *Shulchan Aruch* cites the opinion of the Maharil that an hourglass is *muktzah* because measuring is not permitted on Shabbos. Measuring time, although it is not a tangible item, is nonetheless problematic. This would make the hourglass a *kli shemelachto l'issur*, an item whose primary use is forbidden on Shabbos. Such items are *muktzah* and cannot be moved for convenience — only if its place is needed or for a permitted use like a measurement pertaining to a mitzvah. The *Shaarei Teshuvah*, *Mishnah Berurah*, and *Aruch HaShulchan* write that the prevailing custom is to be lenient with watches, for various reasons.

---

96 *Beis Yosef* 307:17; *Shulchan Aruch* 308:50.

97 307:65.

98 308:164.

Listening

Is a stethoscope similar to the hourglass? It would seem that they are very different. The primary use of a stethoscope is to listen to sounds, not to measure them. Therefore a stethoscope is not an instrument of measuring but one of listening. As such, it is not subject to the concerns of the Maharil's hourglass. Just as a telescope improves our vision, the stethoscope improves our ability to hear sounds within the human body.

Amplification

There is a prohibition on Shabbos called *hashmaas kol* — to amplify a sound. However, this is only if the sound is being amplified to be heard by others. This was one of the many objections raised to using a microphone on Shabbos.[99] However, Rabbi Moshe Feinstein explained that this issue does not apply to hearing aids. Although a hearing aid amplifies the sound, it is only meant to be heard by the wearer, and therefore it is not an issue of *hashmaas kol* (the question of electricity on Shabbos is beyond the scope of this article). This is true with a stethoscope as well. The sound is only heard by the user and is not an issue of *hashmaas kol*.

Conclusion

- In any situation of *pikuach nefesh*, it is obviously permitted to use any device necessary to save a life.
- According to the Rashba, a stethoscope should always be permitted to be used on Shabbos. As such, it is also not *muktzah* and may be moved even just for convenience.
- Those who are stringent like the Rambam and only involve themselves in the study of Torah on Shabbos should not use the stethoscope on Shabbos for non-diagnostic purposes. As such, it is *muktzah* and cannot be moved for convenience.

---

99 *Igros Moshe*, Orach Chaim 3:55; *Tzitz Eliezer* 3:16:3; see also letter published in *Sichos Mishnas Rebbe Aharon* (Kotler) vol. 4.

- Even according to the stringent approach, any medical need should be considered a *dvar mitzvah* and the stethoscope may be used for that purpose.
- According to the Vilna Gaon, the Rambam would permit a stethoscope even for nonmedical uses. As such, all would agree that it is not *muktzah*.

Stethoscopes with Recording Devices

Are stethoscopes that have recording devices inside them considered *muktzah*? In 1965, Rabbi Moshe Feinstein was asked if an electric blanket is *muktzah*.[100] The issue was that the blanket had an electrical heating element inside of it. Does the electric part make the entire blanket *muktzah*, i.e., a *bosis ledavar ha'assur*? Rabbi Feinstein writes that the electric element is not completely *muktzah* (*kli she-melachto l'issur*) and may be moved for a purpose (*tzorech gufo u-mekomo*). Therefore, the blanket is not completely *muktzah* either and may be moved for comfort, etc. Additionally, it could be argued based on the comments of the *Mishnah Berurah* (311:29) that the *muktzah* status of an item is determined solely based on the item's primary usage. Therefore, on the contrary, since the electric element is part of the blanket, which is a non-*muktzah* item, the entire item is not considered *muktzah*.

We could apply this argument to this stethoscope as well. The recording device is incidental to the stethoscope. It is only there to enhance the stethoscope, which is a non-*muktzah* item. Therefore, this type of stethoscope is not *muktzah*.

---

100 Orach Chaim 3:50.

Section II:

YOM TOV AND FAST DAYS

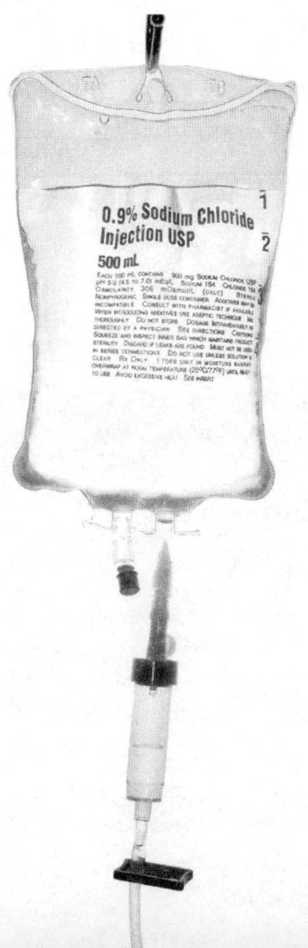

YOM KIPPUR

Using Intravenous to Fast on Yom Kippur

Q: A person must take fluids on Yom Kippur. Should he try to do so through IV, which would not be considered drinking?

A: Although this practice is done in some communities, Rabbi Moshe Feinstein and Rabbi Shlomo Zalman Auerbach raised some interesting objections to it:[101]

The Talmud writes that the Torah needed to give permission for a doctor to heal.[102] One of the explanations why this permission is necessary is because otherwise it could be considered that we are trying to undo a heavenly decree.[103] Rabbi Feinstein wondered if doing a medical procedure, like starting an IV line, not to restore health but to enable a person to fast, is included in that permission. After all, isn't G-d showing that He doesn't want this person to fast? Rabbi Feinstein concludes that there is definitely no obligation to use an IV when "drinking" on

---

101 See *Igros Moshe*, Orach Chaim 3:90; *Shulchan Shlomo*, Refuah pp. 167–168.

102 *Bava Kama* 85a.

103 See *Tur*, Yoreh Dei'ah 336; also see Taz 336:1.

Yom Kippur. Furthermore, he mentions that starting the line for a non-medical purpose may be considered creating an unnecessary blemish.

Rabbi Auerbach was concerned that encouraging such practices undermines the primacy of protecting health. Promoting this type of attitude may discourage people who need to eat from being vigilant to do so. Rabbi Feinstein raises similar concerns.

In summary, according to these opinions, using an IV on Yom Kippur is not necessary or even advised.

Taking Blood Pressure Medication with Water on Yom Kippur

Q: A patient has severe hypertension, but it is well-controlled with a few oral blood pressure pills, typically taken in the morning. May they be taken on Yom Kippur with a small sip of water if taking them without water is not an option? The patient is presently not in danger but the fear is that if they skip their medication, the blood pressure could spike to a dangerous level and potentially be dangerous. Also, would it help to add something bitter to the water, making it taste bad?

A: This question comes up often with various conditions and medications. It can sometimes be difficult to ascertain the level of risk involved if a dose is skipped for a day. Let us present a brief overview:

Future Risk as Risk

In 1966, Rabbi Moshe Feinstein wrote about a situation where the patient needs to take medication for a non-life-threatening condition that could bring on a more serious condition.[104] He ruled that the patient is permitted to take the medication with water if it is necessary. Rabbi Feinstein points out that there is a substantial possibility that a situation of danger could arise from this. As such, taking the medication classifies as *pikuach nefesh*, although it is one step removed.

We could learn this concept from the wording of the *Shulchan Aruch* in the laws of Yom Kippur.[105] There it is written that if the patient has an illness that could worsen as a result of fasting, and that worsened state could bring them to a dangerous situation, they should not fast. It seems that the possibility of a condition deteriorating into something more severe, although a step removed, is already considered *pikuach nefesh*.

Water to Take Medication

With regard to the prohibition of eating on Yom Kippur, medications themselves often are dry and bitter and do not have the status of food. However, people often cannot take them without a sip of water. This complicates matters when it is not clear if this is a situation of *pikuach nefesh*. It is possible, however, that sipping water to take a pill is less severe than regular eating and drinking.

In the laws of blessings, a brachah is not made on water if it is drunk to dislodge something stuck in the throat. The reason is because water does not have taste. Therefore, a brachah is only said if it is drunk to quench thirst, i.e., when there is pleasure from the water similar to taste. However, when water is used to dislodge a piece of food stuck in the throat, it is just being used as an instrument to remove the food. As such, the pleasure is not significant and no brachah is said. Based on this concept, if water is sipped just to swallow a pill, no brachah is said. Here too, the water is only a conduit for the pill.

Following this line of reasoning, we can explore whether water sipped on Yom Kippur solely for the purpose of swallowing a pill violates a Torah prohibition. The *Halachos Katanos* speculates that drinking

---

104 *Igros Moshe*, Orach Chaim 3:91.

105 618.

water on Yom Kippur, even to quench thirst, is not a Torah prohibition. He reasons that water, which doesn't have any taste, is only a rabbinic prohibition. Many authorities disagree with this novel idea and maintain that drinking water for thirst on Yom Kippur does violate a Torah prohibition.[106]

However, we could argue that this discussion is only when water is drunk to quench thirst. As we have learned in the laws of blessings, quenching thirst is a significant pleasure. When the water is solely being drunk to swallow a pill, this is very different. Just as drinking water to dislodge an item stuck in the throat or swallow a pill is not considered a pleasure for the laws of brachos, it may be true for Yom Kippur as well. As such, it is quite plausible that many would agree that drinking water to swallow a pill on Yom Kippur is only a rabbinic prohibition. As such, there may be more room for leniency in cases of need.

Conclusion

Based on these sources we could draw the following conclusions:

- If there is a risk that by missing the dose of blood pressure medication the patient's blood pressure could reach a dangerous level, this is clearly considered a situation of *pikuach nefesh*. Therefore the medication may be taken with water if necessary.
- If missing a dose of medication poses no risk at all, it is not permitted to take it with water. However, it may be permitted to swallow the medicine by itself if it is not in a food-like form.
- If the risks of skipping a single dose of medication are speculative, it is unclear if the patient may take the medicine with water. However, according to our argument that using water to take a pill is not a Torah prohibition, there may be room for leniency.
- According to the *Shmiras Shabbos Kehilchasah,*[107] if the water is made very bitter it may be used to swallow a pill, even for a non-life-threatening illness.

---

106 See *Yabia Omer* 2, Orach Chaim 31:1–8.

107 39:8.

CHANUKAH

Chanukah Candles for a Person with Fear of Fire

Q: An elderly woman lives alone. Years before, she had a fire in her house and has a phobia about having an open fire in her home, to the point that she always goes away for Shabbos in order to avoid having to light Shabbos candles at home. What are her obligations and options with lighting Chanukah candles?

A: In order to fully answer this question, we will explore two points:

- What are the minimal requirements for this mitzvah?
- What is the fundamental structure of the obligation to perform a positive mitzvah when it causes emotional duress?

How Many Candles and Where?

The prevalent custom is to light the number of lights corresponding to the night of Chanukah. However, the minimal requirement is one candle per night. The candle should be lit for half an hour. As such, it would be proper to explore the possibility of lighting a single light, perhaps a *yahrtzeit* candle, for a short period of time after nightfall. This is a complete fulfillment of her obligation, and she may make a brachah on the lighting. Furthermore, she does not need to do the actual lighting. Instead, a neighbor could light the candle and she could still say the brachos.

Attending the Neighbor's Lighting

Does she have the option of going to a neighbor's house for the lighting of the menorah? The Talmud says that the mitzvah of the Chanukah lights is *ner ish ubeiso* — for a household.[108] It is understood that the obligation is to light in a person's place of dwelling. Here are some pertinent points how this concept is developed:

- Many *poskim* conclude that a person does not fulfill his obligation if he lights while traveling in a car, since it is not considered a dwelling.[109]
- A sleepover guest can light where he is staying, since for now this is his place of dwelling.
- Conversely, it is questionable if people visiting family or friends for just a few hours can light there. The problem is that by just visiting, it has not become their place of dwelling.[110]
- A patient in the hospital who has relatives at home fulfills his obligation with the menorah being lit in the home by others.
- Does one fulfill the mitzvah by lighting on a train,[111] or in a wedding hall?[112] There is an argument that although it is not a regular place of dwelling, because one will be there for much of the night, and purchased a ticket or rented the hall, it belongs to them for the time being. Therefore it can be considered their temporary place of dwelling.

---

108 *Shabbos* 21a; *Shulchan Aruch*, Orach Chaim 671:2.

109 *Igros Moshe*, Yoreh Dei'ah 3:14 (paragraph beginning *mi she'ain*); however, see also *Tzitz Eliezer* 15:29.

110 *Shevet HaLevi* 8:158; see *Piskei Teshuvos* 677 for further sources.

111 *Maharsham* 4:146; *Aruch HaShulchan* 677:5.

112 *Piskei Teshuvos* 677:4–5, citing *Kinyan Torah BeHalachah* 5:72.

Based on these sources, we can now examine our situation. It is difficult to assert that going to a neighbor for a short amount of time to light the menorah is a full fulfillment of this obligation. As such, she should not make a brachah if she lights her menorah at a friend's home. However, it is a fulfillment of the obligation of *pirsumei nisa* — to publicize the miracle, to see a neighbor's menorah lit and listen to them recite the brachah of *she'asah nissim*. This is at least a partial fulfillment of the mitzvah.

Electric Menorah

What about an electric menorah? There is much discussion about electric lights concerning the prohibition to kindle a fire on Shabbos, and the obligation to light Shabbos and Chanukah lights.

Many *poskim* conclude that an incandescent bulb has the status of a glowing coal and is considered a fire in respect to the prohibition of kindling a fire on Shabbos.[113] However, they question if it meets the requirements for Chanukah lights. This is because the Chanukah lights are supposed to be similar to the menorah in the Temple. Therefore, it may require a lamp with an actual flame, wick, and a reservoir of fuel. For this reason, many *poskim* conclude that it is questionable if one fulfills one's obligation with an electric menorah. Therefore, it should be lit without a brachah.[114]

Painful Positive Mitzvos

Is she obligated to light the menorah if it will cause her great emotional distress? There are different levels of financial obligation between positive or negative mitzvos. When it comes to transgressing a negative prohibition (*lo saseh*), a person is obligated to give all of his wealth in order to avoid the transgression. However, for a positive commandment, like buying an esrog for Succos, or tefillin, a person is only obligated to give up to a fifth of his wealth.

Rabbi Shlomo HaKohein from Vilna argues that immense anguish is

---

113 *Achiezer* 3:60; index to *Beis Yitzchak*, Yoreh Dei'ah 31; see also *Meorei Aish* by Rabbi Shlomo Zalman Auerbach and *Yabia Omer* 2:26 for extensive discussion.

114 *Be'er Moshe* vol. 6 (*kuntris* electric 58–59); *Yabia Omer* 3:35; *Tzitz Eliezer* 1:20.12.

comparable to giving more than a fifth of one's wealth.[115] Therefore, one is not obligated to perform a mitzvah under such circumstances. Other *poskim* make this point in similar ways.

Conclusion

It would seem that this woman is not obligated to endure great anguish in order to fulfill the mitzvah. However, she should at least go to a neighbor at the time of lighting in order to partially fulfill the mitzvah by seeing the lights and hearing the brachah of *she'asah nissim*.

115 *Binyan Shlomo* 47.

PESACH

Dental Implants, Caps, and Fillings in the Laws of Kashrus and Pesach

Q: A patient asked if they need to change their dental cap for Pesach. What is the halachah regarding dental implants, caps and fillings that come in contact with hot food, both in regard to Pesach and with the laws of milk and meat?

A: Before we begin our discussion, it is important to understand how taste is transferred in the laws of kashrus. Taste is never transferred just through touching alone. The primary method is through heat. However, the level of heat and the method that it is applied can make an important difference in these halachos. We will review some of the early and contemporary discussions about this vexing question.

Early Sources

The advent of dentures spurred a plethora of halachic responsa in the late 1800s on how these devices should be cleaned between milk and meat and for Pesach. The Minchas Elazar of Munkacz had three sets of false teeth, one for dairy, one for meat, and one for Pesach! We will explore some of the different arguments made on the subject, as well as how it relates to the permanent implants of today.

The first argument revolves around the heat of the food normally eaten. If the food normally eaten is not hot enough to transfer taste, there would not be an issue. The Maharsham discusses how hot food needs to be in order to impart its taste into something else.[116] The common definition is *yad soledes bo* — hot enough that a person's hand would recoil if he touched it. One interpretation of this definition is *kreiso shel tinok nichvis bo* — that it could cause a burn to the soft skin of a child. It is possible that adults may occasionally eat foods at this temperature. However, there is an alternative interpretation of *yad soledes bo* that understands it being hot enough to cause a burn to the average adult. Clearly people do not intentionally eat foods that burn their mouths. As such, the Maharsham points out that this difference in interpreting *yad soledes bo* can similarly relate to whether dentures absorb taste.

The Maharsham points out that even if the food is sufficiently hot, whether or not it imparts its taste into the dentures is still subject to another dispute. There is a difference of opinion if taste is absorbed immediately on contact or whether the food must remain on that surface for some duration of time. This therefore also applies to our denture question because hot food quickly passes over dentures and doesn't remain there for a long time.

What emerges from this discussion is that whether or not the dentures absorb taste is subject to two disputes. First of all, this temperature may not be *yad soledes bo*, and second, this momentary contact may be insufficient to cause any transfer of taste. As such, the Maharsham considerers this to be a *sofek sfeika* — a double doubt, and therefore is not a concern.

One of the earliest responsum on this subject, *Shu"t Sheilas Shalom*, gives a different reason to alleviate this concern, suggesting that because false teeth are made of a strong and durable material, they are less likely to absorb the taste.[117]

---

116 1:197.

117 2:195.

Rabbi Shmuel Wosner's Approach

Rabbi Shmuel Wosner in *Shevet HaLevi* makes a very convincing argument.[118] We know that in the laws of kashrus and Shabbos, there is a difference between *kli rishon*, *sheini*, and *shlishi*. The vessel in which liquid was actually heated is called the *kli rishon*, the first vessel. When its contents are poured into another cup, called the *kli sheini*, the heat is less intense than the first, and so too when poured into a third cup, the *kli shlishi*, the heat is even less intense.

In halachah:

- the first vessel, if the heat of the liquid therein is *yad soledes bo*, it can definitely cook and transfer taste;
- the second vessel is subject to dispute;
- the third vessel definitely does not cook or transfer taste, even if it is *yad soledes bo*.
- Many opinions agree that when the contents of the second vessel are poured into the third, the stream going from one to the other already has the lenient status of the third vessel. This is especially true if the stream is interrupted.

With these concepts in mind, the *Shevet HaLevi* analyzes what happens when a person drinks a hot liquid. Rarely does one drink a hot liquid from the vessel it was cooked in, but rather from a soup bowl or cup, which is the second vessel. When the liquid is put into the mouth, it is similar to an interrupted stream because a person doesn't pour the food straight into his mouth. An interrupted stream is like the third vessel that doesn't transfer taste at all! As such, the issue of the dentures is not really that much of an issue at all.

This argument works well for liquids, but what about a solid hot piece of food? The *Shevet HaLevi* addresses a pertinent concept called *davar gush* — a solid item that according to some opinions retains its heat even if it is transferred to a third vessel. However, Rabbi Wosner points out that the Chasam Sofer maintains that this is merely a stringency. Furthermore, it is doubtful if food that is eaten is ever really *yad*

118 1:148.

soledes bo to begin with. As such, Rabbi Wosner concludes that due to the difficulty in koshering the dentures for Pesach, one does not need to be stringent because of the aforementioned reasons.

Natural Teeth

The *Beis Yitzchak*,[119] and *Bais HaYotzer*,[120] make a most fascinating argument that is pertinent to today's permanent dental implants. They ask a most basic question. Our natural human teeth come in contact with hot food all the time and yet we obviously use them for both milk, meat, Pesach and all year round. Why are we not concerned that they absorb meat, dairy, and chometz?[121]

Because of this question, the *Beis Yitzchak* concludes that the food we eat must not be hot enough to transfer taste, and so rinsing one's mouth well is enough to remove remaining particles. Nonetheless, for Pesach, he concludes that if it is not too difficult, dentures should be removed and cleaned with hot water.

Implants, Caps, and Fillings

In our discussion of dentures, some recommended trying to kasher the dentures for Pesach with hot water. This is obviously not possible with permanent implants, caps, and fillings. The argument of the *Shevet HaLevi* is perhaps the most simple and universal. It is especially true with caps and fillings that are on back teeth. Because they are further back in the mouth, they never come into straight contact with liquid because the stream is interrupted by the front teeth and the rest of the mouth. The only question would be with dental implants on the front teeth that possibly come into direct contact with hot liquid from a second vessel. However, as we have learned, there are numerous reasons why food going into the mouth may not transfer taste.

Furthermore, it is quite possible that there is no real question here of a Torah prohibition. As such, it is probable that the rabbis never

---

119 Yoreh Dei'ah I:43:12.

120 See *Sdei Chemed*, Chometz #4.

121 *Shearim Mitzuyanim BeHalachah* 116:4 impressively supports this concept that living materials, like our teeth, can still absorb taste.

placed their restrictions on caps, implants, and fillings that are part of a person's body. Therefore, they should just be cleaned well like a person's natural teeth before Pesach or between milk and meat.

Using Grape Juice at the Seder to Accommodate a Recovering Alcoholic

Q: A recovering alcoholic usually attends a large family Pesach Seder. However, as part of his treatment, he is not supposed to be at an event where alcohol is being consumed. May all the participants at the Seder use only grape juice for the four cups to accommodate the recovering alcoholic, even though wine is preferable?

A: This raises an important and broader question — namely, how much should one person's mitzvah observance be compromised in order to accommodate another person's emotional or physical needs. Here are some sources that could help us draw a plausible conclusion:

A Concerned Relative

Rabbi Shimon Sofer discusses a question pertaining to the mitzvah of succah. A person's relative is very worried about them sleeping in the succah in the cold. They are concerned that it will cause their loved one to become ill. We know that a person who is uncomfortable is exempt from sitting in succah, because the Talmud learns that one is supposed to dwell in the succah like he does in his home, i.e., in a comfortable way. If the person himself is not uncomfortable, but his dwelling will cause his relative to worry and be in discomfort, is this considered a valid exemption from the mitzvah of succah? Rabbi Sofer contends that it is a valid exemption. Just as a person's own discomfort is an exemption from sitting in succah, causing great distress to a relative is an exemption as well. He explains that the reason for the dispensation of discomfort is because it is not the normal way one dwells in one's home. As such, if dwelling in the succah will cause a relative great discomfort, this is also not the normal way of dwelling and he is exempt.[122]

On the surface it seems that Rabbi Shimon Sofer's argument only applies to succah where the obligation is only to dwell in a way people dwell in their homes. However, we do not find people being exempt from other mitzvos because of this dispensation.[123]

A Groom's Anguish

However, the Maharash'dam (1500s) takes this argument further. He permitted a mourner to attend a wedding during the year of mourning [for a parent] if his presence will be greatly missed by the groom. He based this on the halachah that the friends of a groom are exempt from sitting in the succah.[124] He pointed out that one of the reasons given for this exemption is because the friends will be pained by not being able to be with the groom. However, the Maharash'dam understands that this pain is really the groom's pain, which causes his friends pain as well. The Maharash'dam contends that if the Torah obligation to sit in the succah is waived because of the discomfort of the groom, then the rabbinic restriction of a mourner to attend a wedding should certainly be pushed aside to accommodate the emotional pain of the groom.

Preventing Discord

In the 1400s, a widower with children was seeking to remarry. He asked the Terumas HaDeshen if it is appropriate to look for a second wife who is beyond childbearing years. He was concerned that additional half-siblings would cause discord in the family. The Terumas HaDeshen pointed out that having more children than the Torah obligation of a son and daughter is a rabbinic mitzvah, and therefore preventing

---

122 *Hisorirus Teshuvah* 2:21.

123 See *Ohr Sameach*, Hilchos Sanhedrin 15:1.

124 Yoreh Dei'ah #202.

discord is a legitimate reason to refrain from fulfilling this rabbinic precept.[125] However, the Terumas HaDeshen notes that this would not be a sufficient concern to refrain from remarrying altogether.

These sources indicate that in order to prevent the discomfort and emotional pain of others, rabbinic obligations may be put aside. Furthermore, the point could be made that although the Terumas HaDeshen only relied on this dispensation for a rabbinic obligation, it would depend on the gravity of the situation. If there was a serious concern of creating a destructive family feud, which is a serious Torah prohibition of *machlokes* [as the *mussar* teachings of Rabbi Yisrael Salanter remind us], even a more serious obligation could be waived.

Grape Juice at the Seder

There is a discussion if grape juice is just as preferable as wine for the Pesach Seder. While many sources view it as a valid option, Rabbi Moshe Feinstein held that grape juice that has no alcohol content lacks the quality of royalty, *derech cheirus*. Even according to this approach, in a case of necessity, using grape juice or even other beverages is still a fulfillment of the four cups, even though it is not optimal.

Conclusion

The basic rabbinic obligation of drinking the four cups would still be fulfilled even if all the family members drank grape juice instead of wine. It is just less optimal. Therefore, such an accommodation could definitely be made to allow a family member who is recovering from an alcohol addiction to join the Seder.

---

125 1:263.

Mitzvah of Matzo for the Infirm and Elderly

Q: A person must undergo reconstructive jaw surgery sometime over the next few months and will have difficulty eating matzo for the mitzvah in a regular way. Are there ways to make the eating of the matzo easier but still fulfill the mitzvah? If the surgery could be postponed until after Pesach, but will cause great inconvenience, is it permitted to put oneself in a situation where the fulfillment of mitzvos will be compromised?

A: Matzo is usually hard and dry, which can be difficult to eat. In extenuating situations, there are a number of ways that eating matzo can be made easier:

Soaking the Matzo

- The Talmud in *Pesachim* writes that one can fulfill the mitzvah of eating matzo with soaked matzo but not cooked.[126] The reason is because it needs to have the taste of matzo, and the taste changes when the matzo is cooked. However, soaking the matzo for a short amount of time does not alter the taste.
- The Rosh writes that the infirm or elderly can soak their matzo to make it easier for them, as long as it has not become completely dissolved. However, a well person should eat the matzo in the regular way in order not to compromise the taste at all. The *Shulchan Aruch* and Magen Avraham follow this approach.[127]
- According to some opinions it may be soaked in other liquids as well. This is advisable for people who have the custom not to eat

126 41a.

127 Orach Chaim 461:4; Magen Avraham 7.

soaked matzo (*gebrochts*). This is because fruit juice technically does not make flour into chometz — only water. Therefore, eating matzo soaked in fruit juice does not completely disregard this custom.

Determining the Size

- There is a Torah obligation for both men and women to eat a *kizayis*, an olive size amount of matzo, on the first night of Pesach. *Afikomen* according to many opinions is rabbinic, but some contend that it is a Torah obligation (Rashbam). Today, *marror* is a rabbinic obligation because there is no Pesach offering.
- According to Rabbi Moshe Feinstein, a *kizayis* is measured based on the current size of these items. The Talmud states that a *kizayis* is half a chicken egg. Based on this, his son Rabbi Dovid Feinstein, in *Kol Dodi*, measured a *kizayis* as 0.9 fluid ounces, roughly the size of a shot glass.
- In the 1700s, Rabbi Yechezkel Landau of Prague observed a discrepancy between the size of a *kizayis* if calculated as half an egg or the cubic measurements mentioned in the Talmud. For this reason, many *poskim* recommend eating a double *kizayis* for the two times matzo is eaten at the Seder, i.e., Motzi Matzo and *afikomen*, which are Torah obligations. However, Rabbi Avrohom Chaim Noeh contended that there is no real discrepancy between the two. The accepted Sephardic custom also supports this approach. In a situation where eating matzo is difficult, it would seem that the lenient opinions could be relied upon to only eat one *kizayis*.
- The Aruch HaShulchan writes that even if a person cannot eat the amount of matzo and *marror*, there is still a mitzvah to eat as much as possible.[128] However, the brachah on the mitzvah should be omitted.

---

128 477:3.

In summation, here is the list of priorities for extenuating circumstances:

- A *kizayis*, approximately 0.9 fluid ounces of matzo, on the first night of Pesach, is the basic fulfillment of the Torah obligation. The matzo may be ground and soaked briefly in water or other liquids but should not be dissolved.
- According to the Rashbam, a second *kizayis* of matzo for *afikomen* is also a Torah obligation.
- A *kizayis* of *marror* is a rabbinic obligation. If the full amount cannot be eaten, one should eat as much as possible.
- Korech, the matzo and *marror* sandwich, is not a Torah obligation. Because no brachah is said, some maintain that the mitzvah can be fulfilled by eating less than a *kizayis* of matzo and *marror*.[129]

Choosing to Compromise on Mitzvos

According to many *poskim*, a person is not obligated to perform a positive mitzvah if it will cause him to become ill or great pain, even if there is no risk to life.[130] Therefore, a patient who recently had jaw surgery would be exempt from eating matzo if it would cause great discomfort (even if there is no risk of infection). The same would be true for a person with a stomach band who finds eating the full amount of matzo to be very painful.

However, if the surgery could be postponed until after Pesach, is there an obligation to postpone it? This raises a fundamental question with implications to many situations. Is a person permitted to consciously put himself into a situation of duress (*o'nes*) that will exempt him from performing a mitzvah?

Going on a Sea Voyage Close to Shabbos

A classic source often referenced in this discussion is the following halachah:

There is a prohibition to begin a sea voyage within three days of

---

129 See *Sha'arei Teshuvah* 475:1.

130 See *Shu"t Chazon Ovadia* on Leil Pesach for a comprehensive discussion.

Shabbos unless it is for a mitzvah. Rishonim offer various explanations for this restriction. Some write that until three days the traveler is not used to the turbulence at sea and the tranquility of their Shabbos will be disturbed (Rif). Others explain that adverse conditions at sea may require the desecration of Shabbos for survival. As such, setting out to sea so close to Shabbos would make that desecration almost deliberate (R' Zerachiah HaLevi).

It appears from the simple reading of these sources that even if the voyage will *definitely* result in the desecration of Shabbos it is permitted as long as it is for the purpose of a mitzvah or if they departed three days before Shabbos.[131] This halachah seems to indicate that it is not fundamentally prohibited to put oneself in a situation of duress that will exempt one from fulfilling a mitzvah.

The Views of the Toras Chesed and Sdei Chemed

The great Gaon of Lublin in *Toras Chesed* brings this as a support to what he calls a "general halachic principle."[132] He declares that a person is not forbidden from doing something that will lead to a situation of duress where he will be unable to perform a positive mitzvah or transgress a prohibition (i.e,. *pikuach nefesh*). However, it seems that the intent of the Gaon of Lublin was only to be lenient in extenuating circumstances, similar to the case of the voyage that is only permitted for a mitzvah.

In the *Sdei Chemed*, a halachic encyclopedia by Rabbi Chaim Chizkiyahu Medini,[133] there is an entry titled *o'nes haba le'odom al yed'ai atzmo* — the legitimacy of self-imposed duress. The plethora of sources quoted there all maintain that self-imposed duress is not legitimate enough to exempt one from doing a mitzvah. This should lead us to conclude differently from the Gaon of Lublin.

However, it seems that the scenarios of the *Sdei Chemed* and of the Gaon of Lublin are not really the same. The sources quoted by the *Sdei*

---

131 See *Mishnah Berurah* 248:8, 26.

132 2:42:36.

133 *Sdei Chemed* 1, p. 88.

Chemed are referring to a situation where the person *wanted* to be exempt from the mitzvah and therefore engineered a situation of duress. On the other hand, the principle of the Gaon of Lublin is when the motive was never to become exempt from the mitzvah and for other reasons the person enters a situation of duress. For example, the motive of a sea traveler is not to have an opportunity to desecrate Shabbos but to reach a far off destination.

Conclusion

We can now return to our initial question. The patient with jaw surgery is not deliberately trying to make himself unable to perform the mitzvah. The surgery is being done before Pesach for other reasons, i.e., because of the serious inconvenience of postponing it until afterwards. Therefore, based on the principle of the Gaon of Lublin, it would be permitted to undergo the surgery even if the patient may be unable to perform the mitzvah of matzo.

FAST DAYS

Guidelines for Fasting on the Rabbinic Fasts

Q: What are the guidelines for a person who has a non-life-threatening illness regarding fasting on Tzom Gedaliah, Asarah B'Teves, Taanis Esther, Shivah Asar B'Tammuz, and Tishah B'Av?

A: Here is an overview of this very relevant topic:

Basic Sources

The *Shulchan Aruch* writes in the laws of Tishah B'Av that a person with a non-life-threatening illness and a woman after childbirth are exempt from fasting on all fasts except for Yom Kippur because they are of rabbinic origin.[134] The rabbis never made an obligation to fast, even on Tishah B'Av, in a situation of illness. The Rema cites a custom to be more stringent, but concludes that "one who is lenient does not lose."

However, the *Shulchan Aruch* differentiates between Tishah B'Av and

134 Orach Chaim 554:6.

other rabbinic fasts regarding nursing and pregnant women.[135] Nursing and pregnant women are not obligated to fast on Tzom Gedaliah, Asarah B'Teves, and Shivah Asar B'Tammuz, but must fast on Tishah B'Av. Nonetheless, the Rema writes that that there is a custom for pregnant and nursing women to fast on these days if they are not feeling ill.[136]

Taanis Esther

Taanis Esther is less stringent than the other fasts. Therefore, the Rema writes that if a person has a strong headache and is in pain, he does not have to fast.[137] However, he should "redo" the fast at a different date. The *Mishnah Berurah* explains why, if a person is ill, he does not need to fast on a different day when he recovers whereas for a headache he does. He explains an important difference between the two, saying that an ill person has a complete dispensation and therefore does not have to redo the fast at all, but a person with a headache is really obligated to fast, and though we "let him" break the fast now, he must redo it at a later time.

Headaches

The Biur Halachah wonders if this dispensation of a strong headache is limited to Taanis Esther or whether it applies to the other fasts as well. He points out that it may only apply to Taanis Esther, which is not a full obligation. However, the four fasts, which are a rabbinic obligation, should not have this dispensation. Nonetheless, he quotes the *sefer Kovetz* who writes that he saw in the handwriting of "the great Maharaz Emrich, *z"l*," that this dispensation applies to all the fasts. He therefore concludes that each situation should be judged individually.[138]

Defining Choleh

We will now try to achieve a better understanding of these discussions. It is important to point out that the main dispensation for all

---

135 Ibid. 554:5.

136 Ibid. 550:1.

137 686:2.

138 550:1.

of the rabbinic fasts is a person considered to be a *choleh* — ill. The question is then who is classified as a *choleh*?

A person who is sick in bed with a non-life-threatening illness, like the flu, is definitely considered a *choleh*. The Sages viewed weakness as an important concern, even if it is not threatening. Therefore, they did not obligate a person fighting an illness to fast.[139] Along these lines, the dispensation for a woman within thirty days of childbirth is because it is assumed that she is weak and fasting will be detrimental to her health.

For this reason, the *Mishnah Berurah* cites the Pri Chadash, who says that the thirty-day dispensation after childbirth is only if the woman is weak.[140] If she is completely strong then this dispensation does not apply. Likewise, the difference between Tishah B'Av and the other fasts for pregnant and nursing women needs to be understood in a similar way. A pregnant or nursing woman is not ill but rather more vulnerable. As such, the Sages partially considered her to be a *choleh*. For the less stringent fasts, they were therefore lenient but were stringent for Tishah B'Av (unless there is evidence of actual symptoms).

In this light, we can understand the Biur Halachah and *Kovetz*'s uncertainty regarding a strong headache. Perhaps they were grappling with how to view a strong headache that came as a result of the fast. If the person is only experiencing a headache, he is far from being a real *choleh*. As such, such a dispensation could only be applied to Taanis Esther, which is a more lenient fast. Furthermore, one needs to make up the fast at a later date because he did not have the dispensation of being a *choleh*. However, a real debilitating headache that consumes the whole body is quite similar to many other illnesses and could give a person the status of a *choleh*. It is possible that this was the intent of the Maharaz Emrich, who was lenient for a headache on all rabbinic fasts.

Weakness

As mentioned, the Rema cites a custom for pregnant and nursing

---

139 See *Mishnah Berurah* 554:11.

140 Ibid. 554:12.

women to fast even when they are not obligated.[141] The wording of the Rema could indicate that this was not implemented by the rabbis but rather was a custom adopted by the populace. Perhaps this custom evolved because they wanted to be a part of the community and observe these days. As such, the Rema cautions pregnant and nursing women not to be overly stringent and not to fast if they are in pain. He comments elsewhere that "one who is lenient does not lose."

In this vein, the *Chayei Adam* comments on the Rema's words that a *choleh* "does not lose" if he does not fast and that this maxim is definitely correct if one has a weak constitution. Likewise, some write that if the fast will cause a person to feel weak even after the fast, this is an additional reason to be lenient.[142]

Summary

Although situations vary, here are some guidelines based on our discussion:

- Anyone in a life-threatening situation, or even the possibility of one, does not fast on any fast day, not even Yom Kippur.
- A person who is acutely ill with a non-life-threatening condition, such as a fever or the flu, is exempt from fasting on all fasts except Yom Kippur.
- A woman who is pregnant or nursing and does not have her full strength could be lenient with Tzom Gedaliah, Asarah B'Teves, Taanis Esther, and Shivah Asar B'Tammuz. However, if she feels completely fine, she should fast.
- A person with a strong headache does not have to fast on Taanis Esther. If it is very debilitating, he may not have to fast on Tzom Gedaliah, Asarah B'Teves, and Shiva Asar B'Tammuz.
- A person who is not acutely ill but is weak, or has a medical condition that requires him to be careful about preserving his

141 Orach Chaim 554:5.

142 For this reason, in some communities they were particularly lenient on all women of childbearing age regarding fasting. This was out of concern that these fasts would further strain their bodies. See *Piskei Teshuvah* 550, note 5.

strength, may not be required to fast the minor fasts, depending on the situation.

Follow-Up Questions regarding Fasts

Q: a. An ill person needs to eat on Tishah B'Av. Should he try to eat in small amounts with breaks in between, as one does on Yom Kippur?

b. A person with an acute illness such as the flu or fever etc. is not obligated to fast the rabbinic fasts. What about chronic conditions such as Crohn's disease or colitis?

A: Here are some thoughts:

Acute Illness vs. Chronic Condition

There is a basic difference between an acute illness and a chronic condition. One with an acute condition clearly has the classic halachic status of a *choleh kol gufo*, where the entire body feels the illness, or a *nafal lemishcav* — confined to bed.

However, a person with a chronic condition does not notably act different and is even fully functional. Therefore, it is not clear if this has the dispensation of *choleh*. However, arguably these conditions should at least be in a quasi-*choleh* category, similar to pregnant and nursing women. As such, they would be exempt from all the rabbinic fasts except for Tishah B'Av.

Concerning Tishah B'Av, it would be difficult to consider this person a *choleh* unless the symptoms are more concrete. However, if there is a risk that fasting could aggravate the chronic illness, then it definitely has the status of a *choleh*, even with regard to Tishah B'Av. Additionally, individuals who underwent a bowel resection must be particularly concerned with dehydration. The risk of dehydration is definitely considered an illness. In situations where it is unclear, some aspects of the following discussion may be helpful.

Blanket Dispensation

We have mentioned that a *choleh*, an ill person, is not obligated to fast on the rabbinic fast days. The Aruch HaShulchan writes that this is a broad dispensation that completely exempts the ill from fasting at all. Therefore, the *choleh* does not need to eat in small amounts like on Yom Kippur. It has been reported that the Brisker Rav and the Chazon Ish followed this approach. This is also the published opinion of many contemporary *poskim*, including Rabbi Eliezer Waldenberg in *Tzitz Eliezer*, Rabbi Shmuel Wosner in *Shevet HaLevi*,[143] and Chacham Ovadia Yosef in *Yabia Omer*.[144]

In a letter dated the seventh of Av 5669 (1909), Rabbi Avraham of Sochatzov, in *Avnei Nezer*, was asked by his son-in-law, Rabbi Yitzchak Yehudah of Tshechnov, about fasting on Tzom Gedaliah. Rabbi Yitzchak Yehudah had been ill and the doctor advised him not to fast more than midday. Rabbi Avraham responded: "It is clear not to fast at all because in a situation of illness the rabbis never made [it] an obligation."[145] He concludes that this applies to Tishah B'Av as well.

Limited Dispensation

However, the Chasam Sofer, in a responsum from 1811, describes how he became ill on Tishah B'Av of 1811 and needed to drink. He explains that an ill person on Tishah B'Av is only permitted to eat or drink what he needs, and is not exempt entirely from the fast.[146] Similarly, Rabbi Chanoch Henoch Eigash, a justice on the rabbinical court of Vilna before World War II, writes that he was ill and needed to eat on Tishah

143 4:56.

144 10:39.

145 Orach Chaim 540.

146 Orach Chaim 157.

B'Av. However, he ate in small amounts so it could still be considered that he was fasting.[147]

During a cholera epidemic in 1879, the Maharam Shick wrote two responsa about fasting on Tishah B'Av.[148] He writes that one must listen to the doctors and eat and drink however much they feel is necessary to minimize the risks. He adds, however, that it is only permitted to eat how much is necessary, as his rebbe the Chasam Sofer wrote. He also explains the *Shulchan Aruch's* dispensation of a *choleh* more narrowly.[149]

Preventative Measures

The common practice seems to completely exempt an ill person on Tishah B'Av from fasting. This is not like the opinion of the Chasam Sofer and Maharam Shick. It is interesting, however, that the Biur Halachah quotes the work *Pischai Olam* about fasting on Tishah B'Av during a cholera epidemic, who did not give a blanket dispensation to eat, similar to the Maharam Shick but with some different nuances. The *Pischai Olam* writes: "In a place where the epidemic of cholera is not strong, people should eat less than a *koseves* in the amount of time of *achilas pras* as an ill person does on Yom Kippur."

It is surprising that the Chafetz Chaim would quote such an opinion, since in the *Mishnah Berurah* he generally does not require a *choleh* to eat in small amounts. It is possible that the *Pischai Olam* does not usually require a true *choleh* to eat in small amounts on Tishah B'Av as he would on Yom Kippur. Rather, he only endorsed the idea of eating in small amounts when people are well and eating would only be a preventative measure. He is also talking about a situation where the risk of contracting the disease is mild. As such, a distinction could be made between preventative measures and an actual *choleh*. A person who is already ill or who has a high risk of becoming ill already has the status of a *choleh*

---

147 *Marcheshes* 1:14.

148 Orach Chaim 289, 290.

149 It is interesting to note that during the cholera epidemic of 1849, Rabbi Yisrael Salanter publicly ate on Yom Kippur in Vilna. He felt there was an imminent danger and was concerned that fastening would weaken people and make them more susceptible to the disease.

and has a full dispensation from the fast. However, a person who is well and is only preventing illness does not have the full dispensation. Therefore he should only eat what is necessary to avoid the risks. Rabbi Shlomo Zalman Auerbach follows this approach, although the *Yabia Omer* does not make this distinction.

Breastfeeding Mothers

Another situation where this distinction may apply is a breastfeeding mother who may lose her milk if she fasts on Tishah B'Av. She is not ill and does not have the dispensation of a *choleh*. On the other hand, the infant is a *choleh* and it is beneficial for it to have its mother's milk. Some contend that she should eat in small amounts, similar to our discussion about preventative measures.

Summary

Common practice is that someone who is acutely ill or who has a chronic condition that could be aggravated by fasting is completely exempt from fasting on Tishah B'Av. If it is more speculative or preventative, many suggest to only eat or to drink as much as is necessary. This is especially helpful if the patient wants to still be considered as if he fasted at some level.

Section III:

HEALTH, ENDANGERMENT, AND PRACTICING MEDICINE

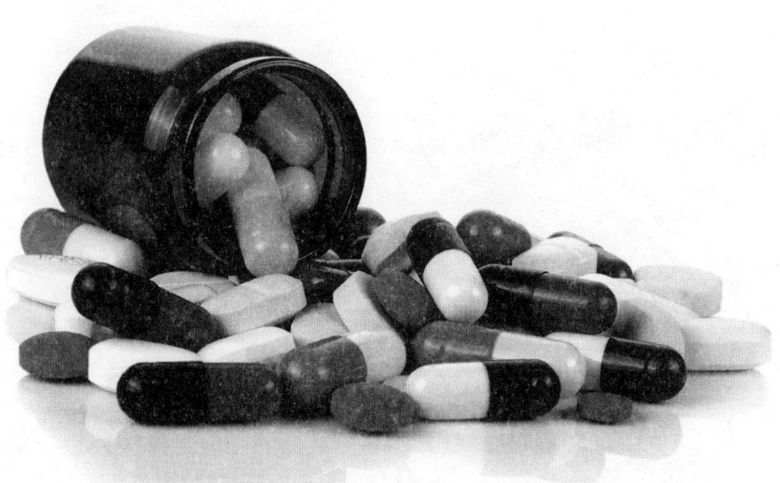

2014 EBOLA OUTBREAK — RISKING YOUR LIFE TO SAVE OTHERS

The 2014 Ebola outbreak in West Africa and the worldwide fear of the spread of the deadly disease raised many halachic and ethical issues, particularly for medical care providers. Are doctors obligated or even permitted to put themselves at risk of getting the dreaded disease in order to save others? We will examine some of the pertinent halachic sources relating to this most serious question.

There are many discussions in halachic literature about epidemics and paranoia over contagious diseases. A few examples:

- In a responsum of Rabbi Moshe Isserles (1500s), he adjudicates a dispute about a landlord who wishes to terminate a rental agreement out of fear of contracting a disease from the tenant's ill wife.
- Rabbi Chaim Palagi (1788–1868) was asked during an epidemic if congregants can stop a physician from attending their synagogue to prevent themselves from being exposed to the contagious diseases that he was treating.
- Rabbi Moshe Shick and Rabbi Malkiel Tzvi Tennenbaum discuss the parameters of fasting during a cholera outbreak in the late 1800s.

Our discussion begins with a responsum of Rabbi Dovid ben Zamra of Egypt (1479–1573), also known as the Radvaz. The Radvaz was asked if a person is obligated to risk his or her life to save another person from sure death. He responded that the ways of the Torah are pleasant and therefore the Torah cannot obligate a person to put his life at risk. While the Jerusalem Talmud indicates that there is an obligation to risk one's life to save another person, most halachic authorities contend that the Babylonian Talmud disagrees. As such, they follow the opinion of the Radvaz that there is no such obligation. This ruling has become a focal point in modern responsa about whether organ donation can be considered obligatory.

The end of the Radvaz's responsum is puzzling, though. He writes that putting one's life in danger, even to save others, is foolish and akin to suicide. Rabbi Ovadia Yosef in *Yabia Omer* cites many sources that disagree with this point.[150] While we do not follow the Jerusalem Talmud's approach that risking one's life is *obligatory*, this does not mean that to do so is *prohibited*. Perhaps the intent of the Radvaz was to highlight a situation where the risks are serious and it is unlikely that it will be successful.

Rabbi Eliezer Waldenberg in *Tzitz Eliezer* deals with our question at length and points out that it is permitted to put one's life at risk to earn a livelihood.[151] He cites two classic examples of this point:

- The *Nodah BeYehudah* prohibited a wealthy baron from going on a dangerous hunting expedition for pleasure but permits such risks to earn a livelihood.[152]
- The *Imrei Eish* writes that it is permitted to enlist in the army as long as the mortality rate is below 16%.[153]

---

150 9, Choshen Mishpat 12.

151 9:17:5.

152 2, Yoreh Dei'ah 10.

153 In 1840, the Imrei Eish was asked if voluntarily enlisting in the army falls under the prohibition of taking one's own life. He responded that it is permitted to take such risks. He proved his point from the fact that in Biblical times, King David took his army out on battles that were nonobligatory even though there was a significant risk of life involved.

Rabbi Waldenberg surmises that if such risks are not significant enough to deter earning a livelihood, all the more so it should be permitted for a doctor to do so to save lives.

There may be an additional dimension to this question. Preventing the spread of a deadly epidemic like Ebola is more than just saving a life, it is about saving society. If not stopped quickly, the epidemic had the potential to kill millions of people and quickly affect the entire globe.

The commentators point out that in the Purim story, Queen Esther put herself in grave danger by appearing before Achashveirosh unannounced. According to the *Yeshuos Yaakov* and *Zichron Yosef*, Queen Esther was permitted to put herself in a situation of certain death because it is permitted to sacrifice one's life to save *all* of the Jewish People. Likewise, Rabbi Waldenberg proposes that a doctor is permitted to put his life at risk to prevent the spread of an infectious disease because saving all of society from a grave risk is of utmost importance.

Rabbi Waldenberg emphatically concludes that a doctor is permitted to treat patients with infectious diseases although he is putting himself at risk. He cites Rabbi Chaim Palagi, who writes that during an epidemic in his city of Izmir, Turkey, the community would hire specific individuals to care for the sick. Rabbi Palagi noted that the majority of the attendants did not become ill, as the verse states: "he who guards a mitzvah will know no harm."

Follow Up Question: Working in a Dangerous Neighborhood

Q: What is the halachic perspective on working as a clinician or first responder in a neighborhood with a very high crime rate?

A: Here are a few thoughts:

- As we have mentioned, the Imrei Eish permitted voluntarily enlisting in the army because the risk to life is less than 16%.

- Furthermore, some point out that although certain areas are considered dangerous, the actual mortality rate is pretty low. This would mean that although shootings and stabbings are unfortunately commonplace in these areas, we must evaluate the risk based on how often clinicians or first responders are hurt, which is ostensibly much lower than the general population.
- We have mentioned that the Nodah BeYehudah permits putting oneself in a dangerous situation for a purpose like earning a living. However, if it is just for recreational purposes, then the commandment of guarding health dictates avoiding such situations.

Conclusion

It would seem that if the actual mortality rate for clinicians and first responders is quite low, then it is permitted, especially if similar employment is not available elsewhere.

Operating on a Jehovah's Witness

Q: A fifty-nine-year-old female patient is scheduled for a liver transplant. As a Jehovah's Witness, she will not accept a blood transfusion, even at the expense of her life. The operation carries a high likelihood of moderate to severe blood loss, which if a transfusion is refused may result in a loss of life. Is it permissible for a Jewish physician to be involved in this operation that may cause the patient to die?

A: The key question here is if operating without the option of blood transfusions is still considered an act of healing or must it be viewed as murder. A few points should be considered:

- We can compare this question to the discussion about the permissibility of risky procedures. For example, a patient is terminally ill but has a chance to survive if a certain procedure is done. Is it permitted to do so if there is a risk that the patient will die immediately as a result of the procedure?
- Many *poskim* conclude that a terminally ill patient may undergo such procedures.[154] They reason that since without intervention the patient could not survive very long (*chayei sha'ah*), the potential for real survival outweighs the possibility of immediate death. According to this approach, the physician's act is considered an act of healing, even if G-d forbid there is an adverse outcome, because the intent was to heal. The fatal outcome is considered beyond the physician's control. However, some distinguish between the levels of risk involved. If the possibility of death is more than 50%, although the intention is to heal, the high mortality rate cannot be ignored.
- Returning to our question, we can assert that the intent of the physician is to heal. Therefore, although there is a risk that the patient will need a transfusion and die, it is still an act of healing and permitted. However, if the risk is above 50%, then it is questionable if it is permitted.
- Another point: if the patient is making a conscious decision to refuse treatment when the need for a transfusion arises, it can be argued that the patient is responsible for her own death.[155]

---

154 See *Igros Moshe*, Yoreh Dei'ah 2:58; *Teshuvos VeHanhagos* 3:356.

155 Another possible differentiation can be made depending on how high the immediate mortality rate is, as opposed to shortly after surgery.

Conclusion

If the immediate risk of death is below 50%, there are strong reasons to assert that it is permitted to perform the surgery.

The Importance of Driving Safely

Tragically, irresponsible driving claims many lives every year. While the prohibition to endanger ourselves or others is well known, people often rationalize their behavior because they don't view it to be so dangerous. This lack of respect for safety regulations can have disastrous consequences. Below, we will present some fascinating halachic sources on the importance of respecting these rules, largely based on a responsum from the late Rabbi Shmuel Wosner.

Maintaining Safe Roads and Preventing Accidents

The Torah tells us to designate cities of refuge to which a person who accidentally murdered can escape. In addition to designating the cities, the Torah writes that it is necessary to "prepare the way." Rashi explains that signs should be posted so he should not get lost.[156] The Rambam writes that this verse requires *beis din* to make the roads straight and smooth and to build bridges over waterways so that he can get there easily.[157] Rabbi Wosner reasons that if we are so concerned for the safety of a person who accidentally murdered, we definitely should have such concerns for the general population. Therefore we are obligated to make our roads safer with traffic signals and speed limits and obviously to abide by them.

An illustration of the importance of public safety is the practice of "pious individuals" mentioned by the Rambam in the laws of torts.[158] Pious individuals would dispose of sharp items like thorns or glass

---

156 *Devarim* 19:3.

157 *Mishneh Torah*, Rotzaich 8:5.

158 Ibid., Nizkei Mamon 13:22.

by burying them deep in their fields to prevent the public from being damaged by them. Likewise, others would incinerate them or throw them deep into the ocean. The lesson is clear — when it comes to public safety, we can never be too careful.

An interesting source that demonstrates the value of preventing accidents is the practice of Rabbi Chaninah recorded in the Talmud.[159] Rabbi Chaninah would fix the roads out of love for the Land of Israel. Rashi explains that he did this so there should not be any accidents, which would cause people to speak badly about Eretz Yisrael. Rabbi Wosner points out that the fact that Rabbi Chaninah chose to demonstrate his love for Eretz Yisrael this way shows the importance he had for preventing accidents.

Respecting Traffic and Driving Laws

In a responsum in *Shevet HaLevi* from 1997, Rabbi Wosner extols communal efforts to raise awareness about safe driving practices.[160] He writes that our obligation to adhere to traffic laws and regulations are more than simply *dinah dimalchusah dinah* — respecting the law of the land. They are a fulfillment of *beis din's* obligation to implement ordinances that protect the public from harm. Rabbi Wosner adds that running a red light, even when no cars are in sight, is forbidden because "it is well known that disturbing traffic patterns brings to danger."

Rabbi Asher Weiss offers a halachic and philosophical analysis of the obligation to respect laws that promote the public good.[161] While there may not be a clear Torah prohibition that one transgresses in a given situation, he argues that it violates a broader moral concept that he calls *ratzon haTorah* — the will of the Torah. This requires us to follow the intent of the Torah's laws, even when there is no clear Torah prohibition. For example, even before the Sages had forbidden activities that detract from the sanctity of Shabbos, there was an obligation to recognize that this behavior was inappropriate. Similarly, the very fact

---

159 *Kesubos* 112a.

160 10:291.

161 *Shu"t Minchas Asher* 2:123.

that the Torah obligates *beis din* or a government to enact laws for the public good demonstrates that the will of the Torah is that we should follow them. Ignoring these regulations, even when there is no foreseeable danger, is disregarding the will of the Torah.

We can learn the importance of uniform standards and practices to promote public safety from a well-documented story about Rabbi Yisrael Salanter. Rabbi Salanter was in Vilna for Yom Kippur during a cholera epidemic. Much to the chagrin of the local *beis din*, he publicly made Kiddush in shul on Yom Kippur and ordered everyone to eat in order that they should not be weak and more susceptible to the disease. Rabbi Moshe Sternbuch offers an interesting explanation of the disagreement between Rabbi Salanter and the *beis din* of Vilna.[162] Presumably, the *beis din* wanted to rule on the matter on a case-by-case basis. Rabbi Salanter felt that it would not be practical. Once some people are fasting while others are not, individuals who should be eating would be hesitant to do so. Therefore, Rabbi Salanter held that the need for uniformity is so great that individuals who may not really need to eat on Yom Kippur must do so.

Conclusion

Torah sources give great value to creating safe roads and preventing accidents in any way possible. Furthermore, it is the obligation upon *beis din* or the local government to enact regulations to ensure safe driving practices. Consequently, it is obligatory for us to follow these rules at all times, even when there is no foreseeable danger.

The Dangers of Texting and Cell Phone Use While Driving

The popularity of cell phones has had some dangerous consequences. Mobile communications are linked to a significant increase in distracted driving, resulting in injury and loss of life. The National Highway Traffic

162 *Teshuvos VeHanhagos* 3:105.

Safety Administration reported that in 2012, driver distraction was the cause of 18% of all fatal crashes, with 3,328 people killed, and 421,000 people wounded in crashes. The Virginia Tech Transportation Institute found that text messaging creates a crash risk twenty-three times worse than driving while not distracted. In most states, texting or cell phone use while driving is illegal. In this chapter, we will explore these issues from a halachic perspective.

Dozing Off behind the Wheel

The late Rabbi Ovadia Yosef and Rabbi Shmuel Wosner both wrote about the liability of a driver who fell asleep behind the wheel and caused serious injuries to the passengers.

Rabbi Yosef discusses a case where Reuven got a ride with Shimon to Haifa. Shimon had hardly slept the night before and dozed off while driving and got into an accident. Reuven was seriously injured and needed to be in the hospital for a month. He then sued Shimon in *beis din* for medical expenses and loss of work.

Rabbi Yosef considers whether the driver dozing off is closer to *o'nes* — beyond his control and therefore exonerated of any fault, or *p'shiah* — negligence and culpable. Rabbi Yosef explains that there are many opinions who generally maintain that a person who unexpectedly dozes off and causes damage is not responsible because he cannot control his body. However, he invokes the Talmudic concept of *techila'so b'p'shiah v'sofo b'o'nes* — that a person whose negligence brought on a situation where the damage was beyond his control is still liable. Similarly, when the driver dozed off, it was obviously unintentional and beyond his control. However, getting behind the wheel with the knowledge that he had not sufficiently slept the night before is clearly negligent. Therefore, based on this concept, the driver's dozing off is viewed as negligence.[163]

A ruling of the Ohr Zaruah, an important Rishon, supports this approach. The Ohr Zaruah ruled that a watchman who fell asleep on the job and allowed the item he was to be guarding to be stolen is

163 *Yabia Omer* 9, Choshen Mishpat 5.

considered negligent and liable. He explains that while falling asleep may be uncontrollable, the watchman knew that his job was to be awake and should have sufficiently slept before. Similarly, both Rabbi Yosef and Rabbi Wosner point out that the driver should have also made sure to have sufficient sleep before getting behind the wheel. Therefore, he is considered negligent and is liable for damages.[164]

Unintentional Homicide

The Maharil writes about a tragic incident where a woman mistakenly smothered her baby during her sleep. He maintains that allowing the infant to sleep next to her is "close to intentional homicide."[165] The Chasam Sofer explains that although the woman falling asleep is not controllable, she should not have kept the infant next to her. For this reason, if the mother took the child to her bed to feed him and fell asleep as she was caring for the child, she is not at fault and does not need atonement. This is because she was doing the best she could do to care for the child.

This ruling of the Maharil demonstrates the same point made in the previous discussion. While falling asleep may be out of a person's control, it is only if the situation was unavoidable. However, if a person has the ability to avoid the situation where falling asleep could cause damage or death, he is fully responsible for his actions.

Distracted Driving

These concepts certainly apply to distracted driving. If a driver becomes distracted because of conditions beyond his control and gets into a fatal crash, it could be considered an *o'nes* and he is not responsible for the loss of life or the damages. However, by picking up a cell phone or texting, the driver is knowingly putting others in a potentially dangerous situation. For example, the National Safety Council (NSC) estimates that speaking on a cell phone while driving reduces focus on the road by 37%. The Virginia Tech Transportation Institute demonstrated that when sending a text while traveling at fifty-five miles per hour, the

---

164 *Shevet HaLevi* 8:301.

165 Shu"t 45.

driver travels the length of a football field ostensibly blindfolded. As such, a fatality resulting from such distraction is close to an *intentional* homicide because he created the dangerous situation. Additionally, because these practices are illegal in most states, the driver is forewarned that these behaviors are really dangerous. Therefore the driver is fully responsible for any resulting death or injuries.

Conclusion

We have demonstrated that ignoring the state laws and texting or talking on the cell phone while driving puts others at risk and is consciously creating a dangerous situation. As a final thought, the Torah writes: "You shall not put blood in your house." The Talmud learns from here that it is prohibited to have dangerous animals or a shaky ladder.[166] Similarly, we find that a person whose animal killed a person is punishable by "death at the hands of Heaven" for allowing this to happen. Rabbi Chaim Brisker points out that this demonstrates that there is a Torah obligation to make sure not to cause monetary or bodily harm. Clearly texting and talking on the phone while driving violate these prohibitions.

Current Halachic Perspectives on Smoking

Q: Is it permissible to smoke cigarettes? Or is it at least a requirement to make a concerted effort to stop smoking?

A: Here are some facts to consider in answering this question:

- Smoking is the leading cause of preventable mortality in the world.

166 *Bava Kama* 46a.

- Over 6,000,000 deaths are directly attributable to smoking annually, 400,000 in the US.
- Up to 50% of all smokers will die of smoking-related illness.
- Most of the deaths are due to cardiovascular disease (heart attacks), chronic obstructive pulmonary disease (COPD), and cancer.
- In addition, smoking contributes to the development of diabetes, the frequency and severity of infection (pneumonia, influenza), and osteoporosis.

Given these types of statistics, in recent years some of the most respected contemporary rabbinic authorities have expressed their serious concerns with smoking, yet the public still seems to be uninformed of these developments. I hope this will provide some up-to-date material on this most important issue.

Rabbi Shmuel Wosner on Smoking

The venerable Rabbi Shmuel Wosner of Bnei Brak, in the volume of his responsa printed in 2002,[167] clearly presents his position on these issues. Here is a summary of his main points:

- The Rambam lists various behaviors, foods, and beverages that Chazal deemed dangerous and prohibited. According to the Ritva, eating these harmful foods is a Torah prohibition.[168]
- The Chasam Sofer cites this Rambam and makes an analogy to the ceremony of *eglah arufah*. This ceremony was performed when a person was found dead between two cities and it cannot be ascertained who was the killer. The leaders of the community closest to where he is found recite a confession whose essence is that "our hands did not spill this blood." The Talmud understands this to mean that the elders are asserting that they could not have prevented the person's murder. Based on this comparison, the Chasam Sofer writes that there is an obligation for community leaders to take an active role in public health and

---

167 *Shevet HaLevi* 10:295.

168 *Shavuos* 27.

safety, "because if the leaders do not do this, then all the blood that is spilled as a result of this inactivity is like they spilled it, Heaven forbid."[169]

- The dangers of smoking are universally accepted and cigarette smoking causes hundreds of thousands of deaths annually and many serious health problems. Therefore, it clearly falls into the category of the Rambam, Ritva, and Chasam Sofer's comments.
- "Therefore, it is clear that according to halachah it is completely prohibited to begin to smoke in the teenage and young adult years, and it is a complete obligation for parents and educators to prevent it."
- "Anyone already accustomed to this bad behavior should make every effort to curb this behavior."
- "Heaven forbid to smoke in public places where others could be harmed."
- "Because, as mentioned, this behavior is tremendously dangerous, publications should not feature advertisements promoting smoking… and anyone who could avoid facilitating smoking is obligated to do so according to the Torah."

Rabbi Dovid Feinstein on Rav Moshe's Position about Smoking

Recently, a scholarly rabbinic journal called *Koveitz Plaitas Sofrim* featured an article quoting the position of Rabbi Dovid Feinstein, the eldest son of Rabbi Moshe Feinstein, on smoking. It addresses a long-held misconception that the concept of "*shomer pesaim Hashem*" applies to smoking. "*Shomer pesaim Hashem*" literally means that G-d guards fools(!). It is used in halachah as a justification for putting oneself in a situation of far-fetched danger. Some people are under the erroneous impression that it could still apply to smoking, given the facts we know today.

---

169 *Avodah Zarah* 30.

In a responsum from 1964,[170] Rabbi Moshe Feinstein asserted that while smoking is not recommended, it cannot be prohibited based on "*shomer pesaim Hashem*." In a later responsum from 1981,[171] under the assumption that only a small percentage of smokers die, Rabbi Moshe Feinstein takes a harder position on the issue but still asserts that if people get great pleasure from smoking, and not doing so gives them pain, it is recommended to stop but is not forbidden. Rabbi Moshe Feinstein's son, Rabbi Dovid Feinstein, makes it clear that his father's ruling was only based on the knowledge of the early 1980s. Since it is clear today that the mortality rates from smoking are extremely high, to use "*shomer pesaim Hashem*" as a basis for leniency has absolutely no basis. This is because any clear danger is halachically forbidden; only negligible risks can be overlooked.

Social Smoking

Here are some thoughts of my own: Most smokers start smoking as teenagers and young adults, usually on an occasional or social basis. While they have heard of the risks of smoking, they either believe that they will not get addicted or will be able to stop. From the limited reading that I have done on teenage social smoking, my understanding is that about a third of social smokers become addicted. In addition, teens are more susceptible to addiction than adults and may actually be addicted without even knowing it. Furthermore, addiction works differently for different people and while some may be able to stop, others cannot. Given these facts, the question becomes is it permitted to smoke occasionally when it may cause an addiction?

The Talmud in *Bava Basra* states that a man may pass a river where women are washing clothing and are not dressed properly for business purposes.[172] However, if he has the option of taking an alternate route and he doesn't do so, he is called a *rasha* — wicked. The reason is that

---

170 *Igros Moshe*, Yoreh Dei'ah 2:49.

171 Ibid. Choshen Mishpat 2:76.

172 57b.

although it is technically permitted if there is no other option, it is forbidden to carelessly put oneself in a situation of temptation. This is true even though it is doubtful whether that person will have improper thoughts by just passing by the river.[173]

We can learn from here a general idea about the concept of *sofek*, using uncertainties to mitigate the seriousness of a prohibition. Uncertainties are only a mitigating factor if a person finds himself unintentionally in that situation. This is why it is permitted to pass by the river if there is no other option. We do not need to assume that he will have improper thoughts. However, it is forbidden to carelessly place oneself in such a situation. For this reason, if there is an alternate route, the person is considered a *rasha*.

We can apply this idea to smoking as well. Smoking has serious health risks, and once a person is addicted it is very difficult to stop. As such, it is forbidden to behave in a way where there is a significant chance it will lead to addiction. As we learned from the case of the river, the fact that there are uncertainties only helps if the person was put in that situation unintentionally. However, it is forbidden to knowingly put oneself in a situation of temptation even if there is a likelihood that one will be able to resist temptation. Accordingly, it is prohibited to begin a damaging behavior that carries with it the risks of addiction with the intention to eventually stop, since for many it is very difficult. As such, it is prohibited to put oneself into such a situation in the first place. This is especially so with health issues where there is the concept of "*chamira sakanta maisura*," that danger to life is more stringent than transgressing a Torah prohibition, and "*ein holchim benifashos achar harov*," that the rule of majority does not apply to a risk of life.[174]

---

173 See also *Igros Moshe*, Yoreh Dei'ah 2:59.

174 Being that susceptibility to addiction varies from person to person, there is a technical reason the doubt concept cannot be used to justify social or occasional smoking that may lead to addiction. If a person is predisposed to easily becoming addicted, for that person the probability of him going from being an occasional smoker to becoming addicted is much higher than the general population. However, he is just not aware of this predisposition. There is a concept of "*sofek machmas chesoron yediah*" — a doubt based on a lack of knowledge, which is not considered an acceptable doubt in the laws of *sfeikos* (see Shach, Klalei Sfek Sfaikah in Yoreh Dei'ah 110). Based on this concept, because each person does not know his susceptibility to

Teen Smoking

The issue of teen smoking, though, is much more complex than a simple lack of education. It has much to do with having a positive self-image and self-confidence, which are crucial in resisting peer pressure. Here are a few examples of how the Talmud requires us to prepare and empower our children for the challenges of life.

In the days of sea travel, the Talmud obligated a father to teach his son to swim so he will be able to swim ashore if he got shipwrecked.[175] Similarly, the Talmud instructs *beis din* to advise a young woman not to marry an old man because she will not have fulfillment in the marriage.[176] Furthermore, we are obligated to avoid placing our children in a situation of weakness and temptation. For example, the Talmud prohibits striking an older son because it is considered like placing a stumbling block in front of him, since he will be tempted to strike back.[177]

The point is that it is the responsibility of parents and educators to do their utmost to provide their children with an environment that fosters their positive emotional and physical well-being in all areas, and certainly free of confusion and mixed messages.

Conclusion

Based on what we know today about smoking, it clearly falls into the category of risks to health forbidden by Chazal. According to many sources, such behaviors violate a Torah prohibition.[178] As such, it is clearly forbidden to take up this practice and one is obligated to make every effort to stop it. In addition, according to my understanding, behaviors that have a significant risk of leading to addiction are inherently forbidden, regardless of whether the person ends up quitting or not. Furthermore, it is our obligation to educate and empower our youth to resist falling into such practices.

---

addiction, he must assume that he is highly susceptible and may become addicted very easily and likewise will have great difficulty quitting.

175 *Kiddushin* 29a.

176 *Yevamos* 44a.

177 *Moed Katan* 17a.

178 See Yoreh Dei'ah 116 and *Darkei Teshuvah*.

Writing Criticism in a Medical Journal and Lashon Hara

Q: Does writing a critique of a colleague's opinion in a medical journal present an issue of *lashon hara*?

A: Here are some points related to this topic:

- Rabbi Yaakov Kamenetsky was asked if it is an issue of *lashon hara* for an editor to write a book review that criticizes an author's work. Rabbi Kamenetsky asserted that the editor is permitted to express his opinion of the book, even if it is critical, because when an author publishes a book for the public, he expects that it will be critiqued. Therefore it is considered that the author gave permission for people to express honest criticism. This is even more so when the author submitted the book to the editor to be reviewed.[179]
- Rabbi Waldenberg of Shaare Zedek hospital addresses two similar questions.[180] Is there an issue of *lashon hara* for a doctor to write a memo that contains criticism of a resident physician's conduct? Similarly, how is it permitted for a doctor to give a patient's medical records that contain confidential information to a secretary to type and file, since the secretary will become aware of the information? Rabbi Waldenberg explains why both of these practices are permitted by using a similar approach as Rabbi Kamenetsky. The resident knows that the physician he is working under will assess his conduct. Likewise, a patient knows that the doctor needs a secretary to assist him with the records. As such, by putting themselves in these situations, they are giving permission for the information to be disclosed in this limited way. Therefore, it is not an issue of *lashon hara*.

---

179 *Emes LeYaakov* on *Shulchan Aruch*, Choshen Mishpat, note 25.

180 *Tzitz Eliezer* 20:52.

However, the secretary is obviously prohibited from disclosing this information to anyone else.

- The logic of Rabbi Kamenetsky and Rabbi Waldenberg should apply to our question as well. Published studies and opinions are presented to the medical and scientific community for their analysis and critique. As such, expressing an honest critique is permitted.
- A final thought: the Rambam defines *lashon hara* as speech that is derogatory or damaging.[181] Expressing a differing point of view in a well-balanced and tactful manner isn't necessarily derogatory or damaging. Furthermore, even derogatory remarks are permitted if it is for a constructive purpose. Therefore, if the author honestly feels that the medical community is misinformed, it is definitely considered a constructive purpose to critique, and therefore it is permitted.

Treating Parents

We will discuss a few questions related to giving medical treatment to parents and grandparents:

Giving Injections to Parents

Q: Is a child allowed to give a parent insulin injections or to test a parent's glucose?

A: Here are some interesting points:

- The Torah prohibits a child from inflicting a wound that draws blood from a parent. The *Shulchan Aruch* writes that even for

181 *Mishneh Torah*, Deios 6.

a medical purpose, a child should get someone else to do it. However, if no one is available, then the child may do it himself. A reason given for this hesitancy is because perhaps the child will injure the parent more than necessary.[182]

- There is also a discussion if whether the parent wanting the child to perform the procedure completely absolves the child from the prohibition.[183] Another contemporary discussion focuses on if there are others available, but their service requires paying a fee, is that considered enough of a reason to be considered "no one available"? Furthermore, to what extent must a person go to find someone else?[184]
- It would seem that a procedure or surgery where there is definite blood loss and significant room for human error should not be performed by one's child unless there is a very substantial reason. The same could be said about starting an IV if the child may have to do multiple pricks in order to get a vein.
- However, a more uniform procedure like testing glucose has less of a chance of error. Furthermore, regular injections do not necessarily cause immediate bleeding and even if so the bleeding is not intentional. As such, if it is inconvenient to have someone else give the injections on a regular basis, there is room for leniency.

Giving a Grandparent Injections

Q: What is the halachah regarding a grandchild administering a weekly injection to a grandparent?

A: This most important question is not directly discussed by the classic sources. The following is primarily based on a responsa of the famous Ben Ish Chai of Baghdad:[185]

---

182 See Yoreh Dei'ah #241.

183 *Minchas Chinuch* #48.

184 *Shulchan Shlomo*, Refuah 2, pp. 263–267; *Minchas Yitzchak* 1:27.

185 *Shu"t Torah Lishmah* #265.

The underlying question is whether or not a grandparent has the status of a parent in respect to the prohibition of causing a wound. The Ben Ish Chai analyzes the various ways grandparents are and are not considered like parents:

- Grandchildren are considered children in regards to the mitzvah of procreation (*peru u'revu*).
- Regarding the prohibition to curse a parent, the *Sefer HaChinuch* writes that a grandparent is not the same as a parent.
- When discussing the mitzvah of honoring parents, the Rema cites the opinion of the Maharik that there is no special obligation to honor a grandparent. However, he disagrees, and bases his disagreement on a Midrash.

Based on these sources, the Ben Ish Chai suggests that a prohibition to injure a grandparent would only be of rabbinic nature. As such, when the intent is to heal it can be permitted. We can add that this is especially true when the question is about an injection where there is little chance of error and may not even cause bleeding. As such, it is permitted to give one's grandparent injections.

Performing a Bloodless Procedure on a Parent

Q: Is it permitted to perform a procedure on a parent that does not involve bleeding but could cause pain, like acupuncture?

A: Let us consider a few important points:[186]

- There is an important discussion between the Rambam and Raavad about the care of parents who are mentally incapacitated, making it impossible for their children to care for them in a respectful manner. The Rambam writes that it is better to leave the care to

186 See *Be'er Moshe* 1:70:10.

others than to care for the parent in a disrespectful manner, while the Raavad questions the practicality of leaving the care to others.[187]

- The *Yam Shel Shlomo*, a classic halachic commentary on the Talmud, tries to reconcile the differences between the Rambam and the Raavad. He contends that both agree that if satisfactory care is available, it is better for the child to leave the care to others. However, when that is not the case, the parent's safety and care are more important than respect.
- It is important to note that there is an obligation to act respectfully to a mentally incapacitated parent who may not even realize or understand what is going on. This seems to indicate that a child has an obligation not to disgrace a parent regardless of the parent's feelings. However, there is a halachic discussion if the parent forgiving his or her honor or pain removes the child's obligation. This would seem to contradict our previous assumption. Nonetheless, there may be a distinction between a parent forgiving the obligation to show respect and permitting actual disgrace. While a parent has the right to waive his honor, disgrace may be different. Disgrace is not dependent on the parent's forgiveness but rather the child's personal obligation. Furthermore, the sincerity of the waiver in such situations may be questionable.

Based on these ideas, it would seem that if the pain is minimal and the procedure is not demeaning, we can assume that the waiver is sincere and it is permitted. Acupuncture should fall into this category. However, if the procedure causes a lot of pain, like setting a broken bone, or demeaning, like inserting a catheter, it is questionable if the waiver helps and should not be done unless it is absolutely necessary.

187 *Mishneh Torah*, Mamrim 1:10.

Dealing with a Patient's Guilt

Q: A patient is suffering from guilt about wrongful behaviors in his past. How should a Jewish practitioner comfort the patient?

A: Here are a few points on this sensitive question:

- The primary issue here is the prohibition of *chanifah. Chanifah* literally means flattery but is essentially referring to condoning wrong actions. To tell a person who sinned that he did nothing wrong violates this prohibition.[188]
- After the Holocaust, Rabbi Yitzchak Yaakov Weiss was asked by survivors, who under that shadow of death aided in euthanasia, about dealing with their past. Rabbi Weiss chose to focus on the extenuating circumstances that these people were in, rather than making an analysis of the permissibility of such actions.[189] He made two interesting comparisons:
  The Rema writes that if a person, out of anger, does an action that is not sanctioned by halachah to a person who abused him, he is not legally responsible.[190] This is because it is considered that he acted under duress. The Rema differentiates between whether or not there was enough time for the person to calm down. Later commentaries are unclear exactly how to gauge this time period. In a similar vein, a person who damages while intoxicated may not be fully responsible for his actions. Rabbi Weiss writes poetically that these survivors were "intoxicated" by their horrible predicament. While he does not write that their actions were permissible, he eases their burden by recognizing how difficult these situations were.

---

188 See Rabbeinu Yonah in *Sha'arei Teshuvah* 3:187; *Igros Moshe*, Orach Chaim 2:51.

189 *Minchas Yitzchak* 6:55,56.

190 Choshen Mishpat 388:7.

- A similar approach is taken by Rabbi Shlomo Wolbe in his fascinating analysis of psychiatry and halachah.[191] Rabbi Wolbe writes that halachah recognizes that feelings of guilt are very debilitating and unproductive. He carefully draws the line between recognizing the difficulty of a situation as opposed to fully condoning the actual behavior.

We can conclude therefore that the primary issue is not to condone the person's behavior by saying it was not wrong. However, it is permitted to recognize the difficult situation that the person was in when he acted this way. Therefore, instead of saying, "Given your situation you did the right thing," the practitioner should respond, "You must have been in great pain if you acted that way."

Hilchos Yichud — Patient Exams, Vision Screening, Home Care

Q: *Yichud* is the prohibition for a man and woman to be secluded together. Here are some important *yichud*-related questions:

- Is a male doctor permitted to close the door to an exam room with a female patient or vice versa?
- Is there an issue of *yichud* when doing vision screening with students in a room with the door closed?
- How can *yichud* be avoided regarding home care? For example, a female nurse tending to a patient when the patient's daughter is going on vacation and only the son-in-law and baby are in the home?

191 *Beshvilei HaRefuah* vol 5.

A: Let us begin with a crash course on some pertinent halachos of *yichud*:

- The *Shulchan Aruch* writes that if there is an "open door" to the public domain, there is no prohibition of *yichud*. There is a major discussion whether an "open door" means that the door is actually open or just not locked. It is questionable whether the open-door leniency works at night or when the people in seclusion are overly friendly with each other.
- Rabbi Moshe Feinstein understands that since today in cities people generally keep their doors closed but open right away when someone they know rings the bell, a closed but unlocked door still has the status of an open door.[192] Regarding the question of whether the "open-door" leniency applies at night, Rabbi Feinstein seems to assert that if there are people on the street at all hours of the night then it would help. He writes further that if there are inner areas in the house, but they are somewhat visible through an open window, this also mitigates the issue of *yichud*.
- In another place, Rabbi Feinstein discusses the practice of many G-d-fearing women who visit a male doctor (or vice versa). He explains that since other patients are waiting for the doctor, or at least there are other staff members in the office, then the doctor is not able to spend an indefinite amount of time with each patient. This fact could mitigate the issue of *yichud*. Similarly, in a hospital setting where other medical staff may come in and out of the exam rooms, this could also alleviate the issue of *yichud*.
- The leniency of having a spouse in the same city may also help in these questions.

Based on these sources, we can generalize that in order for a situation to be considered *yichud*, there needs to be a certain level of privacy and lack of oversight.

---

192 *Igros Moshe*, Even HaEzer 4:65.

Doctor's Visits and Vision Screening

As Rabbi Feinstein mentioned, the doctor cannot spend an indefinite amount of time with a patient. This is because other people are in the office and were the doctor to take too long, someone will page him or knock on the door, which he is then expected to open. Such a situation can therefore be considered as if the door is "open." The same could be said about doing vision screening. For one, the students are expected back into class after the exam, and also, in a school setting, if something is needed from the room other staff members will knock and expect the door to be opened. Therefore, vision screenings in a school would also have this leniency of the "open door."

Home Care

The question about home care is more complicated. If a RN provides homecare in a house that is in a highly populated area, with the door unlocked and the shades open so that an occasional passerby can at least see somewhat into the house, this should substantially mitigate the issues of *yichud*. On the other hand, if he or she is providing care late at night in a quiet suburban area and the house is barely visible from the street, there is a much more serious issue of *yichud*. Such circumstances could be rectified if there are neighbors who could be asked to occasionally come by at all hours of the night, especially if it is feasible to leave the door at least partially opened. However, this may be impractical and therefore such situations of home care are not recommended.

Final Point

Finally, note that the Talmud writes that there is no watchman for inappropriate conduct. This means that we can never be too careful to avoid situations that may lead to wrong behavior. While the laws of *yichud* give a general structure, each person needs to use his good sense to judge when a situation is questionable. Interestingly, the verse states that Devorah, the great judge of Israel, would judge under a date tree. The Talmud explains that she chose this open location in order to avoid any issues of *yichud*.

Pikuach Nefesh vs. the Prohibition of Yichud

Q: In a situation of *pikuach nefesh*, is it permitted to treat a patient if there is an issue of *yichud*?

A: We will examine if the dispensation of *pikuach nefesh* applies to the prohibition of *yichud*:

- According to many sources, one man and one woman being secluded together (if they are not blood relatives) constitutes a Torah prohibition of *yichud*.
- As discussed above,[193] the three cardinal sins (idolatry, murder, and immorality) are the only prohibitions that are not pushed aside for *pikuach nefesh*. The Talmud understands that lesser forms of these cardinal sins maintain this stringency and would *not* be pushed aside for *pikuach nefesh*, meaning that lesser forms of these three cardinal sins are also to be avoided at all costs, even the pain of death. This concept is known as *abizraihu*.
- Rabbi Avraham Yaakov Horowitz of pre-World War II Poland asserted that *yichud*, which is a safeguard to immoral conduct, should also have the stringency of *abizraihu* and therefore be prohibited even in a situation of *pikuach nefesh*.[194]
- Many contemporary halachic authorities, however, maintain that in order to be considered *abizraihu*, the lesser form of the transgression must have some similarity to the actual cardinal sin.[195]
- As such, regarding *yichud*, if the seclusion is intended for immoral reasons, then in that situation it would get the severity

---

193 Page 33.

194 *Tzur Ya'akov*, cited in *Otzar HaPoskim* 22:1–7.

195 Rabbi Y. Roth in *Emek HaTeshuvah* 6:513; *Otzar HaPoskim*, ibid. See also *Igros Moshe*, Even HaEzer 1:56.

of the actual cardinal sin.[196] However, when the intent is clearly to treat an ill patient, and the practitioner is bound by certain codes of conduct, the actual situation does not have any element that would align it with the cardinal sin. Therefore, although such a situation violates the Torah prohibition of *yichud*, if there is no other option, *pikuach nefesh* would take precedence, just as non-kosher food can be eaten in a case of *pikuach nefesh*.

196 *Emek HaTeshuvah* loc. cit.

SECTION IV: MENTAL HEALTH

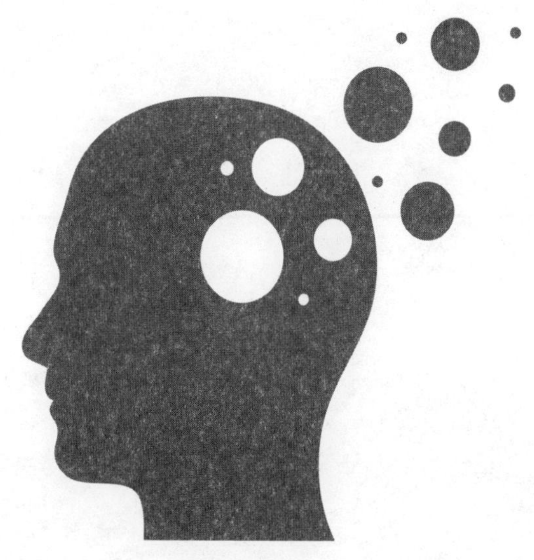

Mental Capacity in Halachah

Q: How does halachah define mental competence and incompetence?

A: A person's obligation in mitzvos, responsibility for actions, ability to give a *get*, *chalitzah*, or to conduct legal transactions all require mental competence. Defining mental capacity in halachah is a fascinating and complex topic. It has been the subject of both modern and age-old rabbinic responsa and was the central issue of the famous Get of Cleves controversy in the 1760s. We begin our discussion of this subject with a passage from the Talmud in *Chagigah* and the conflicting rulings of the Rambam and Rabbeinu Avigdor.

Rabbeinu Avigdor's Approach

The Talmud asks: "Who is considered a *shoteh* (insane)? One who walks alone at night, sleeps in the cemetery, and tears his clothing."[197] Another definition given there is "one who loses what is given to him." Rashi and Meiri understand that these definitions are the criteria for mental competence in all areas: obligation in mitzvos, accountability for actions, and transactions.

In the 1200s, there was an important correspondence between Rabbeinu Avigdor and Rabbeinu Meir about a *get* from the town of Wurzburg. Rabbeinu Meir was concerned that the *get* may be invalid because the husband was mentally unstable. Rabbeinu Avigdor validated the *get* by narrowly interpreting the above passage from *Chagigah*. He

197 *Chagigah* 3b.

maintained that a husband is only considered incompetent if he exhibits the specific behaviors mentioned in the Talmud. Otherwise, even if the husband displayed other abnormal behaviors, he is still considered competent.

Rambam's View

On the other hand, the Rambam (1138–1204) offers a very expansive characterization of a *shoteh*.[198] He writes that "a *shoteh* is not necessarily a person who walks about unclothed, breaks dishes, and throws stones. Rather, anyone whose mind is unstable (*tiruf*) and is always confused about a specific matter is considered a *shoteh*, even if he speaks sensibly about other matters." The Rambam clearly does not limit the classification of *shoteh* to the behaviors illustrated in the Talmud.

Both views — the limited view of Rabbeinu Avigdor and the expansive view of the Rambam — present many challenges. Limiting the definition of a *shoteh* to one who demonstrates the specific behaviors mentioned in the Talmud precludes most mentally ill individuals. While this view may allow a psychotic husband to give a *get*, it would also hold him responsible for his actions. Conversely, in the view of the Rambam, any delusional person would be incapable of giving a *get*, executing a transaction, or bearing responsibility for his or her actions. Either extreme would seem to lead to huge halachic problems.

Maharit on the Rambam

Rabbi Yosef ben Moshe Trani, the Maharit (1568–1639) was one of the first to address the far-reaching implications of the Rambam's position. The brother of a deceased husband came before Rabbi Trani to perform *chalitzah* to permit the widow to remarry. The brother was of minimal intelligence and had slurred speech. Rabbi Trani ruled that the brother had sufficient intelligence to perform *chalitzah*, which doesn't require the same level of understanding as testimony. In his discussion he makes a crucial point about the view of the Rambam, saying that it is possible that the Rambam's expansive view of a *shoteh*

198 *Mishneh Torah,* Testimony 9:9–11.

is only in respect to testimony, but not regarding giving a *get*, *chalitzah*, or executing a legal transaction. According to this approach the Rambam could agree with Rabbeinu Avigdor to a lower standard of mental capacity required for a *get* but would consider such individuals to be incompetent in other areas.

The Get of Cleves Controversy

In the 1760s, an intense rabbinic controversy ensued over a *get* given in the city of Cleves, Germany. It had many historic and halachic implications. At the heart of this controversy was the question how halachah defines and establishes mental competence, and through the various opinions of the halachic authorities involved, we will see how this case helped form the definition of halachic mental competence.[199]

Historical Background

On the third of Elul, 1766, in Mannheim, Prussia, Yitzchak Newberg married Leah Gunzhausen of Bonn. That Shabbos, Yitzchak took the gold coins of his dowry and ran away. He was found in a nearby town, emotionally distraught and claiming that he must flee from the Rhineland. It was suggested that the couple should reside in Bonn until Yitzchak regained his composure. On Friday the seventeenth of Elul, they arrived in Bonn. That Saturday night Yitzchak, in a private conversation with a distinguished relative, insisted that he must leave the country and does not want to leave his wife an *agunah*. There was no *beis din* in Bonn and the couple traveled to Cleves to obtain a *get*. Rabbi Yisrael Lifshitz, the *av beis din* of Cleves, spent hours with Yitzchak and he appeared completely normal. The *get* was given on the twenty-first of Elul, 1766.

Yitzchak's parents did not find out about the divorce until after the *get* was given and their son had fled to England. Understandably, they

199 Fortunately, vast amounts of the original correspondence were preserved in the *sefer Ohr HaYashar* and other works.

were incensed and suspected the Gunzhausen family of foul play. They turned to Rabbi Tevel Hess, the *av beis din* of Mannheim, to annul the *get* on the grounds of mental incompetence. On the fourth of Tishrei, Rabbi Hess and nine other rabbis from Mannheim wrote to the saintly Rabbi Avraham Abish and the famous *beis din* of Frankfurt-on-the-Main to annul the *get*. The *beis din* of Frankfurt maintained that the *get* was invalid and instructed Rabbi Lifshitz of Cleves to comply with their position. When he didn't, they issued a *cherem* and a huge controversy ensued.

The famed Rabbi Yaakov Emden was then in England and examined Yitzchak Newberg and found him to be fully competent. Rabbi Yosef Steinhart, the author of *Shu"t Zichron Yosef*, wrote an important responsum on the subject and concluded that the *get* was valid. In Nissan of 1767, the legendary Rabbi Areyh Leib, author of the *Shaagas Aryeh*, also wrote a responsum affirming the validity of the *get*. Subsequently, Rabbi Yechezkel Landau of Prague, the Nodah BeYehudah, wrote a long responsum validating the *get*. He pleaded with the *beis din* of Frankfurt to explain their reasoning. A year passed and the *beis din* of Frankfurt persisted in declaring the *get* invalid. On Tzom Gedaliah of 1767, Rabbi Yechezkel Landau publicly announced in his sermon that Leah Gunzhausen is permitted to remarry. Nonetheless, the controversy continued until the passing of Rabbi Abish of Frankfurt, on the eleventh of Tishrei 1768. His position remained vacant until 1772, when Rabbi Pinchos HaLevi Horowitz, the author of the *HaFlaah*, assumed the rabbinate of Frankfurt-on-the-Main.[200]

Positions of the Leading Rabbis

On the upside, this celebrated case opened intense discussions about mental capacity in halachah. It is important to understand that while the vast majority of rabbis of the day considered the *get* to be valid, they were far from unanimous in their reasoning.

---

200 This unrest came at the heels of the dispute between Rabbi Yaakov Emden and Rabbi Yehonasan Eybeshitz in the aftermath of the false messiah, Shabtai Tzvi. Many historians believe that these two controversies severely diminished the esteem of the rabbinate and, sadly, possibly allowed the *haskalah* to take a strong foothold.

- As we mentioned previously, according to the opinion of Rabbeinu Avigdor, a person is not considered a *shoteh* unless he exhibits the exact behaviors mentioned in the Talmud. Yitzchak Newberg suffered from a delusion that he could not remain in Bonn and had to flee, but he did not exhibit any of the specific behaviors mentioned by the Talmud. However, the Rambam considers any person with incompetence even in one area of thought as a *shoteh*. The opinion of the Rambam, also cited in the *Shulchan Aruch*, was seemingly the basis of the *beis din* of Frankfurt-on-the-Main's decision to consider Yitzchak Newberg incapable of giving a *get*, thus disqualifying it.
- The Nodah BeYehudah, though, validated the *get* even according to the Rambam by differentiating between the laws of testimony and the laws of divorce. For testimony a person must be of complete sound mind. However, for a *get*, minimal understanding is enough. (This was later the opinion of Rabbi Moshe Feinstein as well.) According to this approach, Yitzchak's compromised mental capacity may have been an issue for testimony but was definitely sufficient for a *get*.
- Rabbi Yosef Steinhart, the Zichron Yosef, did not agree with this differentiation. Still, he considered the *get* to be valid for a different reason. Yitzchak had not behaved strangely prior to the wedding or at the time of the *get* and was presently of sound mind. Therefore, Rabbi Steinhart maintained that the rules of *chazakah* — a halachic assumption, allow us to assume that he was always of sound mind.
- Rabbi Aryeh Leib, the Shaagas Aryeh, validated the *get* for slightly different reasons. He maintained that even according to the Rambam the abnormal behaviors must persist over a substantial amount of time. Rabbi Aryeh Leib felt that Yitzchak's abnormal behavior was too sporadic to change his status.

Mental Capacity and Obligation in Mitzvos

Q: At what point does mental incapacity exempt a person from mitzvos or punishment by *beis din*?

A: The Talmud often states that a minor or insane person is exempt from mitzvos. This concept has many far-reaching implications. A minor is not obligated in mitzvos and we may not be obligated to stop him or her from doing a transgression. On the other hand, a minor is disqualified from performing functions that require an adult. Likewise, defining whether an adult is obligated in mitzvos or not due to his impaired mental status is a sensitive issue. It may permit us to place him in a nonkosher facility, but would disqualify him from performing functions requiring an adult.

Rashi and Meiri

As mentioned above, the Talmud describes specific behaviors that classify a person as a *shoteh*: "One who walks alone at night, sleeps in the cemetery, tears his clothing, and one who loses what is given to him." According to Rashi and the Meiri, these definitions are the exact criteria for mental incompetence in all areas. These sources equate obligation in mitzvos, punishment, and conducting business to one standard. This could be a great leniency or a great stringency. If we understand that in order to consider a person a *shoteh* he or she must exhibit the exact behaviors mentioned in the Talmud, as was the position of Rabbeinu Avigdor, most cases would not be classified as such. This would make their transactions valid but would also consider them obligated in mitzvos and punishable for their actions.

On the other hand, a more inclusive definition of *shoteh* would have far-reaching consequences. It would invalidate the transactions of many individuals, exempt them from mitzvos, and give them a defense of insanity in *beis din*.

The Rambam's View

The Rambam states that the *shoteh* is an invalid witness because he is not a "*ben mitzvos*." According to a simple reading of the text, the Rambam's inclusive definition of *shoteh* applies to obligation in mitzvos as well. Consequently, the Rambam was referring to both testimony and obligation in mitzvos, as shown above, when he wrote: "A *shoteh* is not necessarily a person who walks about unclothed, breaks dishes, and throws stones, [but] rather anyone whose mind is unstable (*tiruf*) and is always confused about a specific matter is considered a *shoteh* even if he speaks sensibly about other matters." We can learn from the Rambam two important points. Firstly, that a person who is delusional only in one area is still considered a *shoteh*. Furthermore, this definition not only applies to testimony but also obligation in mitzvos. As such, individuals with insanity in only one area are completely exempt from mitzvos and are not punishable for their actions. The Divrei Yosef, Nefesh Chayah, Tzemach Tzedek, and Even HaAzel all concur on this point.

Rabbi Moshe Feinstein's Approach

In 1929, as the Rav of Luban, Russia, Rabbi Moshe Feinstein was asked if a delusional young man who professed to be Mashiach had the capacity to give a *get*. Still in his thirties, Rabbi Feinstein wrote a brilliant responsum almost identical to that of the Nodah BeYehudah nearly two hundred years earlier (during the Get of Cleves controversy) brought above.[201] He points out that the Rambam only records his expansive definition of *shoteh* in the laws of testimony but not in the laws of *get* or acquisition. This indicates that it is limited to testimony, not giving a *get* or legal transactions. Therefore, despite the man's delusion that he is Mashiach, he was still competent enough to give a *get*. Rabbi Feinstein therefore allowed him to divorce based on this understanding of the Rambam and the opinion of Rabbeinu Avigdor.

In the course of this discussion, Rabbi Feinstein addressed the general definition of mental capacity for mitzvos and punishment as well.

---

201 *Igros Moshe*, Even HaEzer 1:120.

He points out that the Rambam disqualifies a *shoteh* from testimony because he is not obligated in mitzvos. Therefore mitzvos are obviously subject to the same inclusive definition of *shoteh* as witnesses (like the previously mentioned opinions). Rabbi Feinstein explains that a person who is mentally incapable of observing some mitzvos due to his delusional state is exempt from all mitzvos. This is because the Torah only obligated a person in mitzvos when he is capable to perform all of them.

The Nodah BeYehudah's View

Although Rabbi Feinstein's approach was similar to that of the Nodah BeYehudah, it is different in one important point. They differ in their understanding of a *shoteh's* exemption from mitzvos. While they both hold that the Rambam's expansive definition of *shoteh* in the laws of testimony does not apply to transactions and *get*, Rabbi Feinstein however, like most Acharonim, understands that this expansive definition applies to exemption from mitzvos as well. This means that a semi-*shoteh* is exempt from all mitzvos, even though he can fully perform many of them. On this the Nodah BeYehudah disagrees. He understands that the Rambam does not mean to exempt a mild *shoteh* completely from mitzvos. He gives a novel explanation, saying that the mild *shoteh* is only exempt from mitzvos pertaining to his area of deficiency. However, in areas of behavior not affected by his malady, he is fully obligated in mitzvos. This semi-obligation in mitzvos is sufficient to disqualify him from being a witness. However, it does not fundamentally exempt him from all mitzvos.

Summary

There are three basic views on when mental incapacity exempts a person from mitzvos:

- Rabbeinu Avigdor: only a person who exhibits the exact

behaviors mentioned in the Talmud, or who is clearly insane,[202] is considered a *shoteh* and exempt from mitzvos (based on Rashi and Meiri that there is one standard for all).

- The Rambam (according to most Acharonim, including Rabbi Moshe Feinstein): a person exhibiting strange behaviors in one area is considered a *shoteh* and is exempt from all mitzvos, even though he or she is competent in other areas.
- The Nodah BeYehudah's understanding of the Rambam: A "mild *shoteh*" is not exempt from all mitzvos but only from ones related to his or her area of deficiency.

Contrasting Shoteh and Pesi

We have spent considerable time defining the criteria of what defines a person as a *shoteh* (insane). In this section, we will explore mental capacity from a different angle. Contemporary *poskim* discuss how to view individuals with mental retardation or limited intelligence.

We correctly invest much time and resources into helping these children become as high functioning as possible. However, as they mature we are confronted with the question whether or not they have the status of adults and are obligated to observe mitzvos. Can they receive an *aliyah* to the Torah? May they be placed in a nonkosher facility? On a theoretical level, the contrast between such individuals, who are often referred to as a *pesi*, with the classic *shoteh*, opens a deeper understanding into our previous discussions.

The Difference between Shoteh and Pesi

We return to the Rambam in the Laws of Testimony. After defining the *shoteh*, he discusses the *pesi*, loosely translated as gullible or lacking

---

202 See *Chasam Sofer*, Even HaEzer 4.

intelligence. The Rambam writes, "Those who are exceedingly unintelligent to the point that they don't recognize simple contradictions are included in the category of *shoteh*." The Sema, an integral commentary on Choshen Mishpat, recognizes a basic difference between the *pesi* and the *shoteh*. The *shoteh* may be very sharp and intelligent in many areas of his thinking, but in his area of deficiency is completely irrational and crazed. On the other hand, the *pesi* simply lacks understanding, but his thinking is not turbulent.

Because of this basic difference, many *poskim* view the *pesi* fundamentally different than the *shoteh*. As we have learned, the Rambam famously held that insanity even in one area of behavior classifies a person as a *shoteh* in all areas. The Oneg Yom Tov argues that this concept is limited to a *shoteh*.[203] If a *pesi* has the understanding to perform some but not all the mitzvos, he is still obligated to do what he is capable of doing. The reason for this difference is that the Rambam felt that when a person is delusional, even in one area of his thinking, it is evidence of deficiency in his entire sanity. Therefore, the Rambam maintained that the *shoteh* in one area must be viewed as a complete *shoteh*. However, the *pesi* has no symptoms of insanity — just a lack of understanding. Therefore, even the Rambam should agree that a *pesi's* deficiency in one area is not considered an issue with his overall mental state. Consequently, this would not exempt him or her from all mitzvos.

Mental Retardation

For these reasons, Rabbi Shlomo Zalman Auerbach wrote that individuals with Down's syndrome are not necessarily exempt from mitzvos. If they understand the basic concept that there is a G-d, Torah, and mitzvos, they have the status of an adult and are obligated in mitzvos. However, in areas where they lack understanding, such as the minutia of *hilchos Shabbos*, they are exempt. On the other hand, if they lack even a basic understanding of Torah and mitzvos, they are

---

203 153.

exempt from mitzvos and have the status of a *shoteh*.[204] Rabbi Moshe Feinstein and Rabbi Nosson Gestetner took similar positions on this question.[205]

Summary

After all these discussions of mental capacity in halachah, we can recognize three basic categories:

- A person who is undoubtedly insane or psychotic, or is of minimal intelligence and does not understand the basic concepts of Hashem, Torah, and mitzvos: such an individual is clearly exempt from mitzvos and is unable to execute legal transactions, including giving a *get*.
- A person who functions normally but suffers from delusions and irrational thoughts in a specific area: according to some Rishonim, he is not viewed as a *shoteh*. If the symptoms are persistent, and express themselves in actual behavior, the Rambam considers such an individual to be a *shoteh*. However, many Acharonim limit this classification to testimony and obligation in mitzvos but consider his legal transaction and *get* as valid. Illnesses like schizophrenia or manic-depressive disorder may be included in this category.
- A person who is of low intelligence, like Down's syndrome, but understands the basic concepts of Judaism: such an individual is obligated in the mitzvos he is able to perform, but is exempt from the ones above his level of comprehension.

---

204 *Minchas Shlomo* 1:34.

205 *Igros Moshe*, Yoreh Dei'ah 4:29; *Lehoros Nosson* 7:121.

Dementia and Obligation in Mitzvos

Q: A patient has Alzheimer's disease, dementia, or delirium. What is his obligation in mitzvos? For example, should he be encouraged to avoid eating on Yom Kippur?

A: There may be many considerations why an infirm individual should not fast on Yom Kippur. Nonetheless, we will examine at what point patients with impaired cognitive abilities are fundamentally exempt from mitzvos. It is clear that confusion and a basic lack of understanding exempts a person from mitzvos.[206] However, it is less clear how persistent and permanent this condition must be in order to change a person's status in regard to general performance of mitzvos. Our discussion focuses on a distinction made in the Talmud between a person who is considered merely "sleeping" and still obligated in mitzvos, and one who is a *shoteh* and therefore exempt from mitzvos. The exact clinical application of the halachic definitions is not entirely clear, but this gives us some frame of reference.

Sleeping or Insane?

The Talmud in *Gittin* discusses the laws of using an agent to give a *get*. The Talmud considers the validity of an agency made by a husband when he was of sound mind but during the writing and giving of the *get* he became afflicted by a transient mental condition called *kurkudaikos*.[207]

The underlying question is if this transient state of *kurkudaikos* is like sleep or whether the person is more like a *shoteh*. If we view the transient state like a person who is sleeping, we can still consider him to be fundamentally sane, and as such the *get* would be valid. On the other hand, if we only view the present state and consider him to be a *shoteh*, the *get* will be invalid.

---

206 *Mishneh Torah*, Eidus 9:9, s.v. *tiruf hadaas*.

207 70b.

- Rabbi Shimon ben Lakish rules that the *get* is valid because it is most similar to a person of sound mind who is just sleeping. He distinguishes between *kurkudaikos* and the *shoteh* by saying that while there is no reliable treatment for the *shoteh*, making his condition a permanent ailment, *kurkudaikos* has a reliable course of treatment. The fact that it can be healed makes it transient and not as significant.
- Rabbi Yochanan, though, rules that the *get* is not valid. Unlike a sleeping person who rises from his sleep without intervention, the person with *kurkudaikos* will remain that way unless there is intervention, making him more similar to a *shoteh*.

Intoxication

The Beis Shmuel, a classic commentary on *Shulchan Aruch*, discusses this question in the context of intoxication. What if the husband became intoxicated after he gave the command to write and give the *get*? The Beis Shmuel ruled that the agency is valid based on this passage of the Talmud, comparing intoxication to sleeping and not insanity. A sleeping person is considered sane because he does not need intervention to return to a state of awareness. So too a person who is intoxicated will also regain alertness on his own and is not considered a *shoteh*.[208] The *Toras Gittin*, authored by Rabbi Yaakov of Lisa, concurs with the conclusion of the Beis Shmuel.

However, Rabbi Yechiel Michel Epstein of Novardok, Lithuania, in *Aruch HaShulchan*, had difficulty with the Beis Shmuel's comparison of an intoxication to sleep. A sleeping individual can be roused at any time, but alcohol does not wear off for a number of hours. For this reason, Rabbi Epstein disagrees with the Beis Shmuel's conclusion and ruled that if the husband was intoxicated at the time of the writing and giving of the *get*, it is not valid.[209]

It seems that the Beis Shmuel and Aruch HaShulchan differ in their understanding of the Talmud's comment that to rouse a person from sleep does not require a *maaseh*, an action.

---

208 Even HaEzer 121:3.

209 Ibid.

- The Aruch HaShulchan understands that in order to be considered sane and just "sleeping," it must be possible for the person to regain alertness at *any time*.
- The Beis Shmuel understands that it is not necessary for the person to be able to become alert right now. As long as consciousness will return naturally in a short time without medical intervention, he is considered sane.

Anesthesia

Rabbi Moshe Feinstein in *Igros Moshe* discusses if a Kohen under general anesthesia has an obligation to avoid ritual impurity.[210] He considers the unconscious Kohen to have the status of sleeping, and not that of a *shoteh*. As such, he is obligated to avoid ritual impurity. Rabbi Feinstein explains that being under anesthesia is not comparable to being a *shoteh*. This is because medical intervention is not needed to bring the person back to consciousness, since the anesthesia wears off on its own.

Rabbi Feinstein was clearly not concerned with the issue raised by the Aruch HaShulchan. The patient under anesthesia cannot possibly be aroused at any time. Nonetheless, because he will regain consciousness without outside help, he is not considered a *shoteh*.

The Chazon Ish's Approach

The Chazon Ish gives a unique explanation why a *get* can be given for a sleeping person but not a *shoteh*. The Chazon Ish is seemingly not satisfied with the simple reason that sleep is insignificant because it will wear off on its own, but offers a new reason, saying that sleep is not a change in *etzem ha'adam* — the essence of the person, but is a known life occurrence. Therefore the command of yesterday is still valid. However, insanity is a change in the *etzem ha'adam*, and his entire ability to give a *get* has become impaired.[211]

The Chazon Ish was seemingly bothered by a basic question: Why can an agent write and give a *get* on behalf of a sleeping person if at the time the person is not alert? For this reason, the Chazon Ish

210 Yoreh Dei'ah 1:230.

211 Even HaEzer 86.

understands that the real reason why a *get* can be given on behalf of a sleeping person is not because he could awaken without intervention, but rather because no real change has occurred to his mental capabilities. Similarly, the actions of a *shoteh* are not necessarily invalid because his condition is incurable, but because his mental capacity is fundamentally insufficient. According to the Chazon Ish, the Talmud's indicators of "lacking action" and "medicine available" are not the fundamental criteria of sanity. Rather they are just indicators and may be limited to the discussion of *kurkudaikos*.

Sleeping Pills

Rabbi Yechezkel Roth, a prominent Chassidic *posek* in Brooklyn, takes an approach similar to that of the Chazon Ish. He writes that even if a person took many sleeping pills or fainted and needs medical attention to be revived, he does not have the status of a *shoteh*. Based on the Chazon Ish's approach, Rabbi Roth reasons that in these situations, there was no real change to the brain, and thus the patient cannot be considered a *shoteh*, regardless of whether medical attention is needed.[212]

This conclusion is the direct opposite of Rabbi Feinstein. According to Rabbi Feinstein, the need for intervention, as mentioned in the Talmud, is the determining factor. As such, if the present condition will not subside on its own, then the patient would have the status of a *shoteh*.

Rabbi Y. Roth, in subsequent volumes of his responsa, addresses the care of the elderly with dementia on Yom Kippur. He references his discussion in the laws of *gittin*, where the determining factor is if there is change to the *etzem ha'adam*. Therefore, determining whether such patients have an obligation to fast (as much as their situation allows) would depend on whether their status is permanent or transient and similar to sleeping.[213]

From these sources, three classifications emerge:

- According to the Aruch HaShulchan, it must be possible to rouse the person at any time, otherwise he is considered a *shoteh*.

---

212 *Shu"t Emek HaTeshuvah* 2:102–3.

213 Ibid. 5:93, 7:41.

- According to Rabbi Feinstein, even if it is impossible to rouse the person in his present situation, but his incapacitation will dissipate on its own without medical intervention, he has the status of "sleeping" and is obligated in mitzvos. If medical intervention is needed, he is considered a *shoteh*.
- According to Rabbi Roth, the condition must be viewed as a fundamental change in the person's mental capacity in order to be considered a *shoteh*. (It is not clear exactly how this would be defined medically.)

Alzheimer's, Dementia, and Delirium

Based on these three approaches, we will attempt to apply these concepts to patients with dementia, Alzheimer's disease, and delirium:

- According to the Aruch HaShulchan, we only need to contend with the present state of mind. Therefore, if a dementia patient is confused and unable to process that today is Yom Kippur, he is not presently obligated in mitzvos. This is regardless of whether he is sometimes alert and coherent. This is comparable to the Aruch HaShulchan's ruling that an intoxicated person has the status of a *shoteh* although the alcohol will subside without intervention.
- According to Rabbi Feinstein, the status of *shoteh* hinges on whether the patient can regain his sanity without medical intervention. If the confusion is persistent, even if it may be reversible (as in cases of delirium), he would have the status of a *shoteh* and is not obligated in mitzvos in that state. (It is possible that Rabbi Feinstein may still consider a patient with mild dementia to be obligated in mitzvos if his state of confusion is not persistent but comes and goes.)
- According to Rabbi Roth, a transient condition generally does not make a person into a *shoteh* and he should be encouraged to fast, if possible. This may be true with delirium, which may not be permanent and does not necessarily involve deterioration

of the brain. On the other hand, a patient with advanced Alzheimer's would clearly have the status of a *shoteh* because there is permanent degeneration of the brain that can even be viewed on a brain scan.[214]

Mental Health and Pikuach Nefesh

Q: A psychiatric outpatient is having a crisis on Shabbos. He is not deemed a danger to himself or others. However, if he becomes hospitalized, it may lead to significant life changes for the patient and his family. Is it permitted to take a telephone call from the patient on Shabbos in order to try to prevent inpatient hospitalization? Would it be permissible to travel by car to the patients' home under these circumstances?

A: The dynamics of the relationship between mental health and the concept of *pikuach nefesh* are challenging. I hope these thoughts are helpful.

Rabbi Moshe Feinstein discusses a psychiatric condition that poses even a small risk of the patient hurting himself or others. He writes that such conditions are considered *pikuach nefesh*. As such, even Torah prohibitions like eating on Yom Kippur or driving a car on Shabbos are permitted. He does not address situations where there is no such risk but there are other long-term effects. The question remains how to approach such situations.

The Talmud gives a number of reasons why it is permitted to

---

214 Some opinions maintain that if there is no issue of *pikuach nefesh*, a *shoteh* should not be fed directly because of the prohibition of *lo sa'chilaim*, but may be fed indirectly.

transgress the Torah in order to save a life. One of the reasons given is because "it is better that Shabbos should be desecrated one time so that the patient will survive and observe many more Shabbosim."[215] Rabbi Shlomo Kluger makes an interesting argument. If there is no risk to life per se, but the person's long-term ability to perform mitzvos will be adversely affected, can Shabbos be desecrated? Based on this concept, Rabbi Kluger contends that Shabbos could be desecrated. The whole basis of *pikuach nefesh* is to allow the person to keep more mitzvos. As such, even if a person's life is not in danger, just their ability to keep mitzvos, Shabbos could be desecrated.[216]

Rabbi Kluger's argument has ramifications regarding our question of mental health and *pikuach nefesh*. Although the patient's life is not physically in danger, his mental and emotional capacity is in great danger, which could greatly affect his ability to perform mitzvos. As such, it may be permitted to desecrate Shabbos to avoid a setback.

While Rabbi Kluger's approach is novel, we could make a similar point from a different angle. The *Shulchan Aruch* discusses whether an ailment that affects only one limb of the body is considered *pikuach nefesh*. It then cites a difference of opinion if a Torah prohibition could be permitted to save the limb, ruling in the end that it is difficult to permit a Torah prohibition to save a limb, but a rabbinic prohibition is permitted.[217] Perhaps we can compare the loss of mental health to the loss of a limb. Just as the loss of a limb is very significant, so too a person's mental health is similarly significant, even though it's a "limb" that isn't visible. As such, rabbinic prohibitions may be permitted. Furthermore, mental health is one of the greatest forms of human dignity, which according to some sources takes precedence over rabbinic prohibitions.[218]

Practically speaking, this has several implications:

- Turning on an incandescent bulb on Shabbos is a Torah prohibition because the filament is considered a fire. However, LED

---

215 Yoma 85b.

216 *Chochmas Shlomo*, Orach Chaim 328:46.

217 Orach Chaim 328:17.

218 See *Divrei Chaim* 1, Orach Chaim 35.

lighting, according to many halachic opinions, is only a rabbinic prohibition. Other forms of using an electric current like a telephone would also only be a rabbinic prohibition.

- Driving a car on Shabbos is a Torah prohibition because pressing the gas pedal is igniting a fire, but riding in a car driven by a non-Jewish person is only a rabbinic prohibition.

Based on our discussion, if there is a risk of the patient physically hurting himself or others, it would definitely be permitted to drive to the patient. However, if there is absolutely no such risk, it would be difficult to permit transgressing a Torah prohibition. However, in a situation of significant mental health risks, a rabbinic prohibition could be violated. As such, a mental health professional could take a phone call from a patient on Shabbos (if the receiver could be picked up in an abnormal way [*shinui*] that would be even more preferable). Likewise, it is prohibited to drive to the patient. However, it would be permitted to be driven by a non-Jew.

Seeking Treatment for Problematic Phobias

Q: A person is unable to perform a mitzvah because of a phobia, OCD, or anxiety. If he or she could reasonably overcome the fear with treatment, would that create an obligation to get help in order to perform the mitzvah properly?

A: In order to develop an approach to this and similar questions, we will seek to reconcile some seemingly conflicting sources.

Conflicting Sources

There are a number of sources that seem to indicate that a person is obligated to do so.

- The Rambam writes in the laws of reciting Krias Shema: "A person whose heart is preoccupied and frantic out of concern for the performance of a mitzvah is exempt from Krias Shema."[219] The reason for the exemption is because the mental and emotional involvement in a mitzvah absolves a person from being obligated to perform other mitzvos. This principle is called *o'seik b'mitzvah patur min hamitzvah*. With this in mind, the Talmud in *Brachos* limits this dispensation to a person who is preoccupied with a mitzvah. However, if a person is preoccupied for a reason that is not a mitzvah, there is no dispensation. In the words of the Talmud: "If a person's ship just sank at sea [and he suffered a financial loss and cannot concentrate], he is obligated to [calm himself and] recite Krias Shema."
- Similarly, Rabbeinu Manoach, a Rishon cited by Rabbi Yosef Karo in *Kesef Mishnah* makes this point more clearly. He writes that "a person who is in emotional distress is obligated to calm his mind in order to perform a mitzvah."[220] These sources indicate that a person in distress is obligated to try to calm himself and alter his emotional and mental state in order to perform a mitzvah properly.
- We find a similar concept with an *itstanis*, a very delicate and sensitive person. Such individuals find it difficult to consume large amounts of food. As such, they are obligated to refrain from eating too much on Erev Pesach in order to fulfill the mitzvah of eating matzo properly. We see that an *itstanis* is obligated to have the foresight to avoid having difficulty fulfilling the mitzvah of matzo at the Seder. He can not simply arrive at the seder and say, "I am exempt from the mitzvah because I am an *itstanis*."

---

219 4:1.

220 *Mishneh Torah*, Tefillin 4:1.

These sources therefore illustrate that a person's obligation in mitzvos includes maintaining the proper state of being in order to perform them. One cannot simply say that his present situation exempts him and he has no obligation to change that.

On the other hand, there are many indications that if a person is exempt from performing a mitzvah in the present situation, there is no obligation to change that.

- Rabbi Moshe Feinstein points out that the Rambam does not present living a healthy lifestyle as an obligation. Rather, the Rambam writes that it is recommended. Rabbi Feinstein asks why maintaining a healthy lifestyle isn't an obligation as much as one is obligated to guard oneself from danger. He explains that lifestyle changes are very difficult for people. Therefore, it is difficult to consider it is an absolute obligation.
- In a similar vein, Rabbi Moshe Feinstein writes that "a person is not obligated to invest money to become wealthy in order to give charity."[221] Likewise, if a person has a doorway, he is obligated to affix a mezuzah. However, there is no obligation to create a doorway to have the mitzvah.
- This approach may be an explanation of an interesting dichotomy found in the laws of repaying a debt. The *Shulchan Aruch* writes that "when the loan becomes due and the borrower refuses to pay, the emissary of the court may enter his home and seize items to repay the loan. This is because repaying a loan is a mitzvah and as with all mitzvos, *beis din* can force a person to fulfill his obligation." The *Shulchan Aruch* adds, though, "we cannot force a person to hire himself out to work and repay the loan."[222] It is puzzling why the mitzvah of repaying a debt doesn't compel the lender to work. Why is it different than seizing valuables to repay the loan? A plausible explanation is because obligation in mitzvos is limited to the person's available assets in his present situation. However, it cannot obligate

221 *Igros Moshe*, Yoreh Dei'ah 3:155.

222 Choshen Mishpat 97:15; see also *Teshuvos HaRosh* 68:10; *Imrei Binah* (Halva'ah 2, Givias Chov 2).

a person to create new resources.

- Likewise, a person is only obligated to spend a fifth of his wealth to perform a positive mitzvah. If this is not sufficient, he is exempt. Generally, there is no obligation to solicit money to fulfill a mitzvah (aside from a few exceptions).

These sources indicate that a person's obligation in mitzvos is limited to the constraints of his present situation. If he is exempt in his present situation, there is no obligation to go to great lengths to change that. As such, if a person is legitimately exempt from a mitzvah due to great anguish or fear, there is no obligation to change the situation.

A Possible Explanation

We have learned from the laws of Shema that there is an obligation to calm oneself in order to fulfill the mitzvah. However, a debt collector cannot force the borrower to work in order to repay the loan because he does not have a lean on the person's body. Therefore, a person is not obligated to change that condition to facilitate performing a mitzvah.

Nonetheless, this does not seem to be an inherent contradiction. Fundamentally, the Torah only obligates a person to do what is possible in his present situation. However, if it is not very difficult to come to that state of being, it is still considered within his present situation. As such, there is an obligation to do so.[223] However, if doing so is very difficult, this can no longer be considered part of the present situation. Consequently, he would not be obligated to go through such great pains to change the situation. With this approach we could easily reconcile the discrepancy between the two groups of sources:

- Taking a few moments to calm oneself from a distressing situation in order to recite Krias Shema may not be very difficult. Likewise, in the case of the *itstanis*, it is not very difficult to refrain from eating too much on Erev Yom Tov. Therefore, it

---

223 For example, if a person's tefillin are in a different room, we don't say that he does not have a pair of tefillin available and is exempt from the mitzvah because they are not directly in front of him.

could still be considered part of the person's present state of being.

- On the other hand, for some, changing their diet and daily routine can be traumatizing. Likewise, hiring oneself out may be a significant lifestyle change.
- Becoming wealthy in order to give tzedakah or making a doorway for a mezuzah is entirely different. There is no present obligation whatsoever, but is really creating a completely new obligation.

Interestingly, Rabbeinu Yonah, in his classic work *Shaarei Teshuvah*, makes a remarkable point about the importance of fulfilling positive mitzvos. He writes: "the obligation of tzitzis is only when a person [already] has a four-cornered garment and is not obligated to go and buy such a garment. However, the Sages say that this person is subject to Divine scrutiny because he did not desire in his heart this beautiful mitzvah and its reward."[224] We can learn from here that even when a person is technically exempt, one should still seek to perform the mitzvah, if possible.

Conclusion

Based on our discussion, the obligation to seek treatment depends on how difficult the therapy is. If it does not take much effort, then therapy may be included in the general obligation to calm oneself in order to perform a mitzvah (as mentioned by Rabbeinu Manoach). However, if the therapy is very distressing, especially if the results are not reliable, it does not seem that there is an absolute obligation. Nonetheless, as Rabbeinu Yonah wrote, it is definitely praiseworthy for a person to address his fears and serve Hashem fully.

---

224 *Sha'arei Teshuvah* 3:22.

Preserving Mental Health: An Introduction

Q: A person is obligated to preserve and restore his physical health. What is a halachic perspective on a person's obligation to preserve and restore his mental health?

A: The Rambam devotes the fourth chapter of Hilchos Dai'os to the obligation of maintaining a healthy lifestyle. When he introduces this concept, he writes: "Having a healthy body is necessary for the service of Hashem because it is impossible to gain understanding of the Creator when a person is physically ill. Therefore, one must distance oneself from things that destroy the body, and become accustomed to things that heal and strengthen."

We can learn from this statement of the Rambam an important concept. It is generally assumed that the obligation to guard health refers to our physical wellbeing, not necessarily our emotional and mental health. However, from the Rambam we see quite the contrary. The entire reason it is important to maintain our physical health is primarily because it affects our mental and emotional state.

With this in mind, the Rambam's instruction to "distance oneself from things that destroy the body, and become accustomed to things that heal and strengthen" most definitely applies to mental health as well. We can infer from the Rambam that there is an obligation to lead a lifestyle that maintains and encourages a healthy emotional and mental state.

On a deeper level, there is a mitzvah to emulate the ways of Hashem.[225] The Sages understood that we emulate Hashem by having good character traits. The Rambam devotes the first three chapters in Hilchos Dai'os to discussing the proper balance between different character traits. Based on this, it seems that a person with serious issues in

225 See *Sefer HaChinuch*, mitzvah 611.

anger management, low self-esteem, etc., has a mitzvah (and possibly an obligation) to seek professional help when it has been shown to be effective. This is especially true if it impacts the lives of others.

Addictive behaviors like alcoholism and substance abuse are serious issues from a halachic perspective for many reasons. Addictions often cause physical and emotional harm to oneself and others. Furthermore, the very concept of addiction goes against the Torah ideal that a person should have self-control over his instincts.[226]

Conclusion

Halachah recognizes the importance of maintaining good mental health and its central role in serving Hashem and maintaining healthy relationships. Therefore, there may be a halachic obligation to seek professional help for mental health issues, just like with physical illness, depending on the severity of the situation and the effectiveness of the available treatments.

Choosing a Mental Health Care Provider

Q: What should a Torah-observant person look for when choosing a mental health care provider? Is this different from choosing a regular doctor?

A: In a letter from 1960, Rabbi Moshe Feinstein writes that religious Jews have always sought medical care from any practitioner regardless of his or her personal beliefs. However, when it comes to counseling, the "remedy" is not a medicine or procedure but rather a personal conversation. Therefore, the personal beliefs of the therapist can play a much larger role than when treating physical

---

226 See *Igros Moshe*, Yoreh Dei'ah 3:35.

illness. He voices concern that the patient may be counseled or directed in a way that may conflict with the observance of halachah, core beliefs, or general sensitivities to a Torah way of life. Therefore, he writes, "one should seek a *shomer Torah* psychiatrist, and if it is not possible, one should get an assurance that he will not speak about faith and Torah with the patient."[227]

Conclusion

Psychology, as a study of human behavior, interfaces with how we think, act, and feel. For this reason, it may come into conflict with Torah values. It is therefore important to seek help from a practitioner that is *shomer Torah u'mitzvos* or at least has a reputation of being respectful of a Torah lifestyle.

Perspectives on Psychology and Psychotherapy

Q: How do Torah sources view the theoretical and clinical aspects of psychology and psychotherapy?

A: This is obviously an open-ended, important, and fascinating question.

Introduction

Rabbeinu Bechaye wrote about secular knowledge: "there is no form of secular knowledge that does not have inaccuracies... however, our Torah is like pure silver without impurities."[228] While this was written

227 *Igros Moshe*, Yoreh Dei'ah 2:57; [regular doctor, Yoreh Dei'ah 4:8].

228 *Devarim* 30:12.

about all branches of secular knowledge, this is particularly important when dealing with psychology. Many of the founders of modern psychology viewed the essence of man and religion in ways that conflict with Torah values. For this reason, contemporary *poskim* are cautious with how these ideas should be implemented.

Theoretical Aspects of Psychology and Psychotherapy

Here are a few thoughts:

- Dr. M. Spero, cited in the Encyclopedia of Jewish Medical Ethics, points out that some psychotherapists view religious practice as an interference with their treatment. He observes that Freud, Jung, and Skinner had issues with the impact of religion on mental health.
- Rabbi Shlomo Wolbe, a great contemporary master of mussar and hashkafah, wrote a masterpiece on the interface between Torah and psychology.[229] He demonstrates that the core of Judaism is *yedidus* — friendship. Judaism is characterized by the warmth and friendship between man and G-d and between mankind. The antonym of *yedid* is *achzar*, which although literally means "cruelty," the word comes from the words *ach zar* — but a stranger. According to Judaism, evil and cruelty come in absence of the warmth of G-d and mankind. Rabbi Wolbe points out that individuals whose beliefs are devoid of this intrinsic relationship between man and G-d are left alone in life, like a stranger. On the other hand, authentic Jewish thought provides a security blanket of warmth, self-worth, and self-esteem. This has great value in combating feelings of depression and self-negation. Many of these ideas were particularly stressed by the founders of Chassidus. Sadly, the early pioneers of psychology, many of whom were unaffiliated Jews, were not exposed to this perception of Judaism. This could have given them a better appreciation for Jewish religious practice.
- Rabbi Wolbe writes that Judaism recognizes the role of the

229 Published in Sanz Hospital's Journal *Shvilei HaRefuah*, vol. 5.

subconscious. He quotes the letters of Rabbi Yisrael Salanter, the founder of the *mussar* movement. Rabbi Salanter encourages setting aside times to study ethical teachings with repetition and emotion. He explains that these exercises will help bring out feelings and yearnings that are buried deep in the subconscious. Rabbi Wolbe points out that Rabbi Salanter had acknowledged the role of the subconscious "sixty years before Freud!"

- Rabbi Wolbe points out that the Sages recognize the existence of mankind's base instincts. However, he criticizes Freud for asserting that libido is the only instinct. Furthermore, Rabbi Wolbe stressed a critical difference between how Rabbi Salanter viewed the role of the subconscious, as opposed to the founders of psychology. While Freud focused on the influence of the subconscious on the conscious, he largely ignored the opposite, i.e., the ability of conscious efforts to influence all levels of a person, which is a primary teaching of Rabbi Salanter.
- The contemporary Chassidic work *Nesivos Shalom* stresses the idea of self-realization. He explains the importance of connecting with a person's soul known as *daas*. Chassidus views the subconscious as a gold mine of potential and spirit, not jealousy and desires.

Clinical Psychology

In a clinical setting, may an observant therapist use methods that do not conflict with halachah but were developed or influenced by psychologists whose understanding of human behavior conflicts with Torah values? Does the method's questionable origin prevent us from utilizing it?

Rabbi Moshe Feinstein wrote: "It is simple that it is permitted to use discoveries in medicine and inventions made by nonbelievers (*apikorsim*) and give them acknowledgment, because it is only prohibited to give recognition to them in areas of holiness, not secular."[230] We see that fundamentally we are permitted to use advancements in secular knowledge regardless of its origins. If the method is "kosher," it is permitted on its own right.

However, when it comes to psychology, it may conflict with Torah thought in very subtle ways. Therefore, the integration of these ideas needs careful study by individuals with a profound grasp of Torah thought. Rabbi Nosson Gestetner advises: "In these matters one should consult a pious Torah scholar who will know what to distance and what to bring close."[231] He also writes that before we assume an approach is appropriate, we should look into Torah sources to find reference to such ideas.

Psychology's Place in Torah Thought

Notwithstanding these concerns, Torah sources acknowledge the value of a secular study of human behavior. Rabbi Salanter writes that character development needs "worldly wisdom," apparently meaning an understanding of human nature and experience.[232] The Rambam famously wrote in *Shemoneh Perakim*, which discusses human behavior, to "accept the truth from anyone who speaks it." This concept, however, needs explanation. When it comes to the study of Torah we clearly do not seek secular sources to advise us. How and when is it appropriate to seek secular sources when it comes to human behavior? Where does the exclusive spiritual realm of the Torah begin?

Rabbi Chaim Vital, the famous student of the Arizal, questions why the Torah does not command directly to have good character traits, and answers that the Torah was given to individuals who are already good and decent people.[233] Good character traits are a prerequisite. This idea could be expressed, based on the thought of the Maharal of Prague, that the purpose of the Torah is not to make bad people good, but good people better, and ultimately perfect.

---

230 *Igros Moshe*, Even HaEzer 1:96, s.v. *ubetzem misupkani*.

231 *Lehoros Nosson* 3:66.

232 *Ohr Yisrael* #2.

233 *Sha'arei Kedushah* 1:2.

With this idea in mind, we could approach the place of psychology in Torah thought. The Torah was given to people with stable emotions and good mental health. As the Rambam writes in Hilchos Yisodei HaTorah that through Torah a person has the ability to perfect himself and reach the level of prophecy. This is the realm of the soul and is exclusive to Torah.[234] However, Rabbi Salanter quoted above was referring to the basic struggle to overcome bad character traits like anger and jealousy. Emotional issues are not exclusively the realm of Torah. Good emotional and mental health is a prerequisite to Torah. As such, the "worldly knowledge" mentioned by Rabbi Salanter may be appropriate to help overcome these challenges.

We can develop this concept further with a unique interpretation of a statement of the Rambam in which he says, "it is a disgrace to use the Torah as a remedy."[235] He explains that the purpose of the Torah is not to heal the body but the soul. Based on the ideas of Rabbi Vital and the Maharal, we can assert that the "healing of the soul" mentioned by the Rambam is not referring to emotional issues like bad character traits, but to man's ability to connect with the spiritual. Healing emotional dysfunction is therefore still within the realm of the physical.

This approach could limit the possible conflict, at least at a clinical level, between Torah beliefs and psychological methods. The Torah sources are primarily addressing individuals with normal emotional function and behavior. However, the role of psychology is primarily to assist individuals with emotional dysfunction.

Rabbi Wolbe, in *Alei Shur*, makes a similar distinction. He writes that the great masters of *mussar* did not dismiss the influence of a person's past on his present behavior. Rather, they viewed the present and future as opportunity for change and development and ultimately influence the subconscious.[236] As such, Rabbi Wolbe recognized the value of the psychoanalytic approach of viewing a person's present state as

---

234 7:1.

235 *Mishneh Torah*, Avodah Zarah 11:12.

236 *Alei Shur* vol. 2, pp. 140, 169.

being influenced by the past. However, he relegates it to the treatment of situations of true abuse and dysfunction.

Conclusion

The clinical use of psychology by a practitioner who is sensitive to halachah and a Torah lifestyle for patients with serious mental anguish and dysfunction is appropriate. However, the integration of various concepts and attitudes of modern psychology in general needs careful discretion. It requires both an understanding of psychology as well as a profound and broad understanding of Torah sources. This can be challenging because unlike regular halachic questions, there may not be a clear approach.

Biological Causes for Human Behavior vs. Free Will

Q: Does it contradict the Torah to promulgate the perspective that human behavior is exclusively or even primarily a function of biological processes? Seemingly such an approach precludes the notion of free will, which is an integral assumption of Maimonides' Thirteen Principles of Faith.

A: The notion that behavior is affected by a biological process may be a modern phenomenon. However, there are some interesting discussions in early Torah sources about the interface between the concept of free will and other factors that Chazal recognized as having an effect on human behavior, e.g., *mazal* — forms of astrology, which cause different tendencies like a predisposition to murder etc. and problematic lineage. Let us review some of the literature on the subject.

- The Talmudic Encyclopedia quotes a responsum from the Geonic period that addresses whether the notion that a person's tendencies are predisposed of by *mazal* contradicts free will. According to the responsum, if it is believed that a person could overcome the predisposition and change his or her behavior, there is no conflict with the concept of free will. However, the belief that a person's tendencies are completely determined by *mazal* and cannot be overcome does indeed contradict the concept of free will, a cornerstone of the Torah.[237]
- In a similar vein, the Meiri, a Rishon, discusses extensively the relationship between *mazal* and free will. He writes that while people are born with certain tendencies, its influence over his life isn't absolute and (with effort) a person can change his behavior.[238] Based on this, he explains the concept of *ain mazal l'Yisrael* — that the Jewish People are not controlled by *mazal*, to mean that although a person is born with certain tendencies based on *mazal*, a person can work to overcome them. The Meiri in his work on repentance discusses these ideas at length.[239]
- Rabbi Yaakov Yisroel Kanievsky, the Steipler Gaon, cites an interesting Radvaz about the character traits of illegitimate children.[240] The Radvaz writes that although according to the Talmud, parents' immoral behavior affects the character of the children, it only means that it is more difficult for them to change but not impossible. Therefore, it is not a contradiction to the idea of free will.
- The Talmud writes that a person born under the "red" *mazal* will spill blood and become a murderer, butcher, bloodletter, or mohel.[241] Rabbi Shlomo Wolbe explains that the *mazal* is only a general disposition to blood, but a person has free will how to channel it. According to Rabbi Wolbe, while a person cannot

---

237 Vol. 2, *itztagninus*.

238 *Shabbos* 156a.

239 See also *Bircas Avraham* on *Shabbos* 156a.

240 *Kehilas Yaakov*, Yevamos.

241 *Shabbos* 156a.

change the underlying disposition, there will clearly be ways to use it in proper and constructive ways.

Conclusion

The classic Torah sources definitely recognize that people may be born with predispositions that make it more difficult for them to control certain behaviors. However, they reject the notion that as a general rule people cannot overcome these obstacles. Furthermore, as Rabbi Wolbe points out, the natural leanings should be channeled in a way that doesn't disregard them, but gives direction within the framework of halachah.

Seeking Treatment for Hurtful Behavior

Q: Is a person with anger management issues or a controlling personality obligated to seek therapy?

A: Here are some points to consider:

- Hurtful behavior is far more serious than simply a lack of altruism. The *Yam Shel Shlomo*, a classic halachic work on the Talmud from the late 1500s, writes: "It is a Torah prohibition to damage another person, even indirectly, because although there is no monetary payment, it violates the command 'You shall love your friend like yourself.' "[242]
- Along the same lines, the Rambam and *Shulchan Aruch* both

242 *Yam Shel Shlomo* on *Bava Kama* 10, 23. In a similar vein, the *Sefer HaChinuch*, mitzvah 243, writes in the commandment to love a fellow Jew: "One who loves his friend like his own soul will not steal his money, overcharge, or unfairly compete with him, and will not damage him in any form."

write that causing embarrassment, even when not subject to monetary retribution, is a grave sin. These sources demonstrate the seriousness of such behavior. It should follow that if there are effective treatments available to better control these behaviors, then the perpetrator is fully obligated to seek them.

- During the tumultuous times of the Dark Ages, the Rambam was asked about the status of Jews who superficially converted to Christianity in order to avoid expulsion and persecution. In Hilchos Yisodei HaTorah, the Rambam wrote: "Everyone is obligated to sacrifice his life rather than transgress the Torah, and one who did not do so desecrates Hashem's name... nonetheless, since it was done under duress, they are not punishable by *beis din*... However if he is able to save his soul and escape from under the dominion of the evil king and does not do so... it is considered that he *deliberately* worshiped idolatry."[243] The Rambam therefore teaches us an important halachic principle: even if a person is in a legitimate situation of duress, if he neglects opportunities to leave or change the situation, his failure to act makes him responsible for his conduct.

Conclusion

Often people with severe personality issues like unmanageable anger, controlling personalities, or a tendency of verbal abuse attribute their disposition to disturbing childhood experiences. While there may be some legitimacy to their claim, there are often effective therapies available that can help them control their behavior and avoid harming others. We can conclude that if appropriate treatment is available, such behavior can no longer be rationalized or excused. They are fully obligated to seek appropriate professional help to avoid the grave Torah prohibition of harming others.

---

243 5:4.

Spousal Abuse, Alcoholism, and Gambling

Q: Can a spouse or family member with an alcohol or gambling problem be compelled to seek treatment?

The destructive effects of a spouse with a history of physical or emotional abuse, alcoholism, or gambling addictions are unfortunately not a new phenomenon. Rabbinic responsa spanning hundreds of years grapple with these most difficult situations.

- In the late 1500s, Rabbi Shlomo Luria vividly describes a husband clearly addicted to gambling and alcohol. In the course of his discussion, he writes, "If [the wife] says he is repulsive to live with because of his depraved ways, as he continually drinks whiskey at their taverns and comes home drunk, and defied his commitment not to gamble and threatens to endanger, burn, destroy, and sell [the assets], there is no greater legitimate claim [for divorce] than this."[244]
- Along the same lines, Rabbi Yom Tov Tzahalon writes of a deplorable domestic situation: "If she despises him because of his deplorable actions, adultery, and frivolity — *yasher koach* (kudos) [to her]!"[245]
- In a case of domestic abuse from the 1200s, Rabbi Shlomo ben Aderes gives the spouse the full right to make an ultimatum about their relationship. He writes: "Her claim to not return to him unless he commits to stop his physical and verbal abuse is correct."[246]

It is clear that these great rabbis viewed behaviors like physical and emotional abuse, alcoholism, and gambling as simply unbearable and inexcusable. It violates the basic obligations between spouses according to the Torah and the mutual commitments of the *kesubah* — the

---

244 *Shu"t Maharshal* 69.

245 *Shu"t Maharit Tzahalon* 229.

246 *Shu"t Rashba* 4:113.

Jewish marriage agreement. As such, it was expected that any form of reconciliation must be accompanied by an unwavering commitment to change these behaviors.

Conclusion

In contemporary times, with the great amount of research done in mental health, abuse, and addictions, we have gained significant understanding of these complex patterns of behavior. There are effective programs available to help overcome these challenges. Based on our discussion, there is a definite halachic obligation for an abuser or addict to seek professional help and rabbinic guidance to satisfy his or her basic family obligations.

Addictions and Self-Control

Q: Is there an obligation for an addict to seek rehabilitation, even if the behavior does not cause harm to himself or others?

A: This question can be analyzed from different angles:

Emulating the Ways of Hashem

The Torah instructs us to exemplify the ways of Hashem. The Rambam understands that we exemplify the ways of Hashem by having pleasant and balanced character traits. The Ohr Sameach, however, points out that the obligation of having proper character traits varies from person to person depending on their capabilities in serving Hashem.[247] In this context, the Rambam writes, "We are commanded to

247 Talmud Torah; see also Mabit in the introduction to *Beis Elokim*.

go in these balanced ways, as they are good and just, as the verse states, 'you shall walk in His ways'... a person is obligated to conduct himself in these ways and exemplify Hashem *according to his ability*."[248]

The *Sefer HaChinuch* says on this issue, "One transgresses this positive commandment by not trying to straighten his ways, conquer his inclination, and perfect his thoughts and actions toward the love of G-d."[249] We can learn from the *Sefer HaChinuch* an important point. As the Rambam wrote, a person is only expected to fulfill this mitzvah to the extent of his abilities. This may greatly depend on each person's mental, emotional, and physical capabilities, and life situation. However, the *Sefer HaChinuch* stresses that we all must try no matter what challenges we face. Completely ignoring this objective is a definite transgression.

Ben Sorer U'Moreh

The Torah speaks of the *ben sorer u'moreh*, the delinquent youth who steals money from his father to buy meat and wine. The Torah prescribes a very severe punishment. The Talmud explains that since he has become accustomed to such habits at such a young age, he will surely become a gangster and will rob and murder and thus "it is better that he should die innocent than guilty." However, the Talmud comments that even though *beis din* never actually gave this punishment, the Torah nevertheless teaches this halachah to tell us the severity of such behavior.

The Ramban, in his commentary on the Torah, asks what transgression the youth actually committed by eating meat and drinking wine or stealing money, none of which are punishable by death! The Ramban answers that his behavior shows a total disregard for the precept of *kedoshim tihiyu* — sanctifying ourselves. Although this great commandment can be fulfilled on many levels, the youth is blatantly disregarding the entire concept. As such, coupled with the eventuality that the youth is likely to murder, this behavior is viewed as most serious.[250]

---

248 *Mishneh Torah*, Daios 1:4–6.

249 611.

250 *Devarim* 21:18.

Rabbi Moshe Feinstein on Drug Addiction

In a letter from 1973, Rabbi Feinstein addresses the many halachic issues with substance abuse. He writes that "It is simple that it is forbidden because it violates many basic Torah principles and is a serious prohibition." In the course of his discussion Rabbi Feinstein raises many issues, such as health risks, causing distress to parents, and a person's obligation to keep his mind clear in order to learn and daven properly. He also cites the comments of the Ramban about the *ben sorer u'moreh*, that the ungirded pursuit of pleasure transgresses the commandment to sanctify oneself.[251]

A most interesting part of Rabbi Feinstein's letter is how he views becoming an addict. He draws a comparison between willfully becoming an addict and the severity of the *ben sorer u'moreh*. He understands that the issue with the *ben sorer u'moreh* is that he is putting himself into a situation where he will lose his self-control. Once he has become accustomed to eating meat and wine, he will do anything to get it, even to steal and eventually murder. Bringing on this loss of control is the severity of the issue.

Therefore Rabbi Feinstein argues that the same could be said about addictions. While an addict may not necessarily steal or murder, he is giving up his self-control by creating a new desire. Rabbi Feinstein writes: "[the addiction] causes a great desire, more than the natural desire for food, which is necessary for a person to live. Once accustomed to these substances, it comes to the point that some people cannot control or remove [their dependency]. This is a serious prohibition, as we find that the *ben sorer u'moreh* is punished for an uncontrollable desire for food although it is kosher. Therefore, it is definitely forbidden to cause an uncontrollable desire for something that there is no need for."

Rabbi Feinstein understands that the severe punishment of the *ben sorer u'moreh* is for creating an uncontrollable desire for something not essential for human existence. Rabbi Feinstein makes a similar point about nicotine addiction for new smokers.[252]

---

251 *Igros Moshe*, Yoreh Dei'ah 3:35.

252 *Igros Moshe*, Choshen Mishpat 2:76.

Conclusion

The Talmud records the fatherly advice of Rav to his son Chiya: "Do not ingest substances."[253] Rashi explains this to mean, "do not become habituated to ingest substances [because] it will become a routine and your heart will ask for it and you will squander money." The plethora of sources cited in this discussion demonstrates the many issues with addiction. As Rabbi Feinstein noted, it is our responsibility to make sure that we do not become needlessly dependent on substances or behaviors. For these reasons, when there is a situation of addiction, we should make use of the many programs and techniques available to curb such behavior.

253 *Pesachim* 113a.

SECTION V: SHIDDUCHIM, PREGNANCY, AND BIRTH

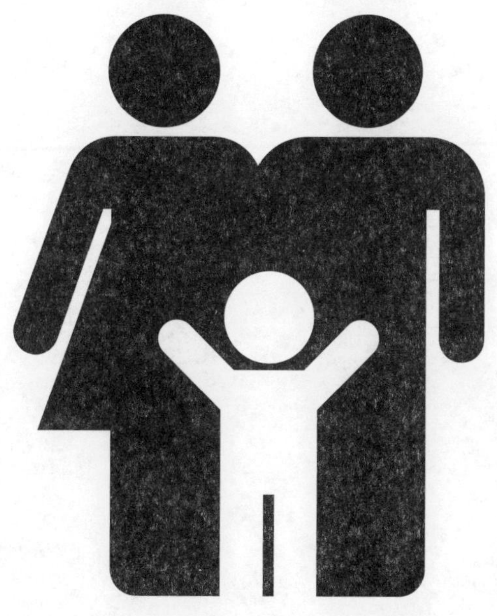

BRCA Mutation and Shidduch Information Disclosure

Q: In recent years, a specific genetic marker has been identified for some occurrences of breast cancer, known as the BRCA gene. The more severe mutation is called BRCA1 and the less severe form is called BRCA2. This has raised many important questions about the disclosure of this information during the shidduch process. In our discussion we will consider the following scenario:

The mother and maternal aunt of a young woman have both battled breast cancer and are carriers of the BRCA1 mutation. The daughter has not been tested and there is a 50 percent chance that she is a carrier. A close friend of the family who is aware of the medical history would like to suggest a *shidduch*. What is the responsibility of the *shadchan* to both parties regarding withholding or disclosing this information?

A: We will begin our discussion with some of the halachic background about disclosing medical information for *shidduch* purposes in general, and then we will focus on its application to this situation.

The "Cherem" to Break a Formal Engagement

Rabbeinu Gershom Meor HaGolah passed away nearly a thousand years ago (d. 1026 CE). He enacted many important *takanos*

— ordinances — that still impact Jewish life today. The most famous one was the *Cherem DeRabbeinu Gershom* officially prohibiting polygamy.

Of particular interest to our discussion is his *takanah* about breaking a formal engagement. Unlike in most communities today, a binding legal agreement was signed at the time of the engagement.[254] This *takanah* was an important improvement because in those times, families made huge financial investments and expenditures prior to a wedding, and a broken engagement could mean financial ruin. Rabbeinu Gershom's *takanah* invoked a *cherem* — excommunication — and a monetary penalty for breaking the commitment without good cause. For the next hundreds of years, rabbinic responsa would seek to define the fine lines of this *takanah*.[255]

In order to appreciate these discussions, we must keep in mind that marriages were commonly arranged by a third party between two families in distant cities. The families would only meet each other (bride and groom included!) when they journeyed to the other town for the wedding. Often there were surprises when they found (or so they felt) the prospective son- or daughter-in-law simply unfit for marriage. A heated battle in the rabbinic courts would often ensue, with one party claiming damages for the other's breaking of the *takanah* and the other claiming they were deceived and that they are the ones entitled to compensation.

In the 1700s, Rabbi Yechezkel Landau in *Nodah BeYehudah* was asked about a family who broke an engagement when they discovered that the prospective bride had very poor hearing.[256] Because it was still before the use of hearing aids or sign language, the only way to communicate with her was by shouting loudly. Rabbi Landau reasoned that the couple would be forced to discuss private matters loudly, which could easily be heard by others. This could be viewed as a serious objection to the match. Therefore, he ruled that this was a justifiable reason to break the commitment.

On the other hand, not every claim was given such sympathy. In the

254 Today *tenaim* are not usually signed at the engagement but at the wedding to avoid this issue.

255 *Hatakanos BiYisrael* by Rabbi Y. Shipansky; also see Rema, Even HaEzer 37:4; *Piskei Teshuvah* (2).

256 1:53.

late 1600s, a family broke an engagement and tried to evade paying the penalties by claiming that the prospective bride's nose was too long (!). Rabbi Yair Chaim Bachrach in *Chavos Yair* dismissed their claim as frivolous. He explained that a *mum* — a blemish — is only significant if it is unusual. Rabbi Bachrach further demonstrated that a long nose is perfectly normal, and proved his point with a concept from the laws of *agunos*. When identifying the body of a deceased husband, a long nose is not considered even a mediocre *siman* — identifying characteristic, because it is so common. Obviously a long nose is common and therefore not a substantial reason to break an engagement. Therefore, he ruled that the groom's claim was frivolous and he must pay full damages for transgressing the *cherem*.[257]

Disclosing Medical Information for Shidduch Purposes

Contemporary *poskim* discuss the permissibility of withholding medical information during the *shidduch* process. They often draw upon the concepts used in earlier responsa about breaking a formal engagement.

Rabbi Moshe Feinstein in *Igros Moshe* deals with a case of a young woman who did not have regular menstrual periods (possibly polycystic ovary syndrome, which is common among Ashkenazim). According to her physicians, she was fertile but may not be able to have many children. The family wanted to know if they are obligated to disclose this information to the other party. Rabbi Feinstein writes that the Talmud implies that in general people are not particular on family size. Therefore, it is not considered a serious blemish and it is not obligatory to disclose this information.[258] On the other hand, Rabbi Meir Bronsdorfer in *Kenai Bosem* considers epilepsy to be a serious blemish because the condition can affect the quality of the couple's life in many ways. For this reason he ruled that the disclosure of epilepsy *is* obligatory.[259]

The common thread between all of these discussions is that in order

257 220.

258 Even HaEzer 3:27.

259 1:121.

to create an absolute obligation of disclosure, the issue needs to have a significant impact on the couple's life in a way that is uncommon in the general population. Long noses and small families are common, but epileptic seizures and communicating solely by shouting are not.

The BRCA Mutation

In order to apply these principals to the BRCA mutation, we will begin with some basic statistics about this mutation:

According to the National Cancer Institute, about 12 percent of women in the general population will develop breast cancer sometime during their lives. However, according to recent estimates, 55–65 percent of women who inherit a harmful BRCA1 mutation, and around 45 percent of women with BRCA2 mutation, will develop breast cancer by age seventy. Additionally, women with BRCA1 have a 39 percent risk of ovarian cancer, compared to the 1.4 percent risk of the general population (BRCA2 11–17 percent).

Together, though, BRCA1 and BRCA2 only make up for 5 percent of all breast cancers.

While there are options of preventative surgery, screenings, and treatments, they are not foolproof (according to one study, the reduction is 50 percent) and the condition can have substantial impact on a marriage.

Are Gene Mutations Considered a "Mum"?

According to the Chavos Yair mentioned previously, a common imperfection or condition is not a legitimate reason to break an engagement.[260] If a problem is common, we can assume that people are not so selective about it and the other party had no reason to disclose it.

The BRCA mutation, though, is clearly unusual. According to one report on genetic testing in Israel, the prevalence of BRCA1 is 1 in 100, and BRCA2 is 1 in 75. This is quite uncommon when compared to Tay-Sachs, which is 1 in 25–30, or Gaucher's disease which is 1 in 7–18. Another indication of this is that statistically BRCA mutations

---

260 220.

only make up 5 percent of all breast cancer, and the prevalence of breast cancer is around 12 percent in the general population. Therefore, a family history of BRCA should fall into the category of a condition that needs be disclosed.

On the other hand, genetic mutations are intriguing. They are not concrete and present conditions, like epilepsy, but rather a more abstract concern that the person has a greater likelihood of contracting a devastating illness. This is especially poignant with breast cancer, where the majority of cases are not related to genetics. One could argue that a mutation is too intangible to be considered a "blemish" at all! Truthfully, however, there is strong halachic basis to assert that halachah views genetic mutations and hereditary conditions as very concrete concerns.

Hereditary Conditions

The *Shulchan Aruch* writes: "One should not marry a woman from a family of lepers or from a family with epilepsy. However, this rule only applies when it has been established three times that their children have had this condition."[261] In the times of the *Shulchan Aruch*, these conditions were considered fatal. Some understand that it is even prohibited to marry under these circumstances. Others raise the question why only three times, and not two, constitutes a *chazakah*. It should be comparable to the halachah that forbids circumcising a child born to a family which lost two children due to excessive bleeding.

The *Chasam Sofer* dismisses the notion that there is a prohibition to marry under such conditions. He disputes the comparison to the laws of circumcision, which forbids the third child in a family whose first two sons died as a result of circumcision from receiving one himself. Since the circumcision is an act performed by someone else, we must take the utmost caution and even consider two times a *chazakah*, as opposed to an illness that comes on its own and is not our doing.[262]

This dialogue clearly demonstrates that the Sages viewed hereditary conditions as serious and concrete. Furthermore, it is possible that

261 Even HaEzer 2:7.

262 137.

there is an obligation of disclosure even when a *chazakah* has not been fully established. We must keep in mind that the requirement of two or three family members needed to create a *chazakah* was said in the context of a possible prohibition to marry, not just when disclosure is necessary. As such, if a family has a significant history of hereditary disease, there should be an obligation of disclosure.

Genetics as Halachic Evidence

Furthermore, we can learn about the relationship between genetics and halachah from the post 9/11 discussions about using DNA evidence to permit *agunos* to remarry. The consensus was to consider DNA as a strong indicator of identity.[263] This conclusion was based on establishing that each person has a unique DNA pattern. This was done by creating the halachic concept of a *ruba de'lesa kaman*, an abstract majority based on samples of the general population (a million people out of a world population of about seven billion). These samples demonstrated that we can assume that each person's DNA is unique. Therefore, DNA is a reliable indicator of identity even for the serious questions of *agunos*. Returning to our discussion, this demonstrates that when properly established, genetics play an important role in halachah.

Unlikely Concerns

Going further, there may even be an obligation to disclose a serious familial issue when the likelihood of it materializing is distant. The *Piskei Teshuvah* cites the Beis Meir's response about a bride who broke her engagement when she became aware that the brothers of the prospective groom were mute. Her concern was that if her husband would pass away childless, she would be unable to receive *chalitzah* from the mute brothers and be left unable to remarry. The Beis Meir considers this to be a sufficient reason, even though the likelihood of this happening is not very great. He explains that although the Talmud says most women become pregnant and give birth, which should lead us to assume that her husband will not die childless (and he may outlive her),

---

263 Possibly a *siman muvhak*. See *Yeshurun* vol. 12 for an extensive discussion.

nonetheless, because many people consider this to be an important concern, the bride has a legitimate reason to break her commitment.[264]

The ruling of the Beis Meir is very significant. It demonstrates the enormity of a devastating but unlikely concern about the future.

Drawing Conclusions about the BRCA Mutation

As we noted, carriers of BRCA1 have a 55–65 percent likelihood of getting breast cancer.

These halachic sources demonstrate that genetic mutations that are likely to have serious future consequences are a legitimate concern. A carrier of BRCA1 has a very high risk of a disease with great impact on the couple's life. Therefore, these factors should be part of the couple's decision to marry.

In our case study, the young woman was not tested and may not be a carrier (50 percent chance). However, the fact that her mother and aunt are carriers may create a *chazakah* that would require disclosure of the family's medical history. When should it be disclosed? Read on.

When Is Disclosure Necessary? Disclosing Previous Transgressions

Rabbi Moshe Feinstein in *Igros Moshe* deals with this question in a letter of encouragement to a young woman who wanted to do *teshuvah* on her promiscuous past. Must she disclose this information to a potential match? He writes that she does not need to reveal it to him during the initial dates, but must do so when they are seriously considering marriage.[265] Likewise, Rabbi Feinstein justifies a young divorcee initially concealing her previous marital status. He explains that even though she is obligated to tell a future husband at some point, she could conceal it until he gets to know her well. By doing so, he will not be deterred by the fact that she was previously married, but were she to reveal this earlier, potential husbands might not even consider the match.[266]

---

264 Even HaEzer 50:5.

265 Orach Chaim 4:118.

266 Even HaEzer 4:32:4.

Concealing Undesirable Lineage

Rabbi Yaakov Yisrael Kanievsky, the Steipler Gaon, in *Kehilos Yaakov*, took this point even further.[267] The Talmud in *Yevamos* relates that a person whose father was not Jewish asked Rav Yehudah how he could find a wife, because people only wanted to marry into fine lineage. Rav Yehudah advised him to flee to a place where his status is not known and find a wife there of reputable lineage.[268] The obvious question is: How could he deceive the people of this far-off country about his personal status?!

The Imrei Yosher suggests that because no one will ever know about his lineage, it makes no real difference.[269] The Steipler, however, advances the possibility that because the objection is more superficial, once the couple is married the past will be viewed as insignificant. At that point, she will readily overlook it. Based on this argument, the Steipler Gaon suggests that a person with a minor halachic question on his lineage does not have to reveal it if later it will be overlooked. However, he concludes that his discussion should not be relied upon as *halachah lema'aseh* — practical halachah.

A serious concern with the Steipler Gaon's approach is that there is a fine line between acceptance and coercion. Ideally, a spouse may be so happy about his new husband or wife that he or she readily accepts certain flaws that were previously unknown. It could be argued that if we know that this is the case, such information could be initially withheld. More often, however, this is not the case. The spouse is simply stuck in his or her situation with no easy way out. He might not readily accept the situation at all and could be the victim of deception.

A Delicate Balance

Rabbi Feinstein's approach of disclosing after a few dates seeks to balance the issue of deception while still letting people have a chance to meet without being stigmatized. Additionally, Rabbi Feinstein

---

267 *Yevamos* 44.

268 45.

269 2:114.

sought to avoid letting damaging personal information become public knowledge. This would be a serious form of *lashon hara*. According to this approach, it is permitted for the couple to begin meeting without disclosing information. However, this is only acceptable as long as there is a possibility that once the other party is made aware of the issue he may overlook it and continue the relationship.[270] This is not considered deceptive because it is normal not to share such information at the beginning of a relationship. However, once it is expected for these issues to be disclosed, they must do so. Continuing the relationship without disclosure is putting the other person in an unfair and painful situation, which is wrong.

In light of this discussion, we can conclude that the family history of BRCA1 does not need to be disclosed before the couple meets. However, when the relationship becomes earnest, the issue of the BRCA mutation should be raised.

The Responsibility of the Shadchan

The *Shulchan Aruch* writes that it is prohibited to give a rubbed-out coin to an unscrupulous merchant because he may use it to cheat others.[271] The Imrei Yaakov postulates that this may be a general concept not limited to coins. As such, he objects to the practice of many *sofrim* — scribes, who sell tefillin and mezuzos with indiscernible mistakes to middlemen, since although these items are only "*kosher be'dieved*," dishonest merchants may end up selling them as "*mehudar*." Just as in the case of the rubbed-out coins, it is the responsibility of the original seller to avoid such deception. However, if the mistake is easily discernible, then it is not the responsibility of the seller.[272]

This line of reasoning could be used in defining the responsibilities of a *shadchan*. As Rabbi Feinstein wrote, it is forbidden to disclose the family's medical history prematurely because it will unfairly become public knowledge. Therefore it would not be the role of the *shadchan*

---

270 Because the couple is not yet engaged and entrenched in the relationship, it can be assumed that if they agree to marry despite this issue it is genuine.

271 Choshen Mishpat 237:18.

272 Ona'ah 10.

to disclose it. As such, generally the *shadchan* can assume that the family will act properly and disclose the information at the proper time. Furthermore, if the family's struggles with breast cancer will come up during the dating process, it may be viewed as a discernible imperfection that is not the responsibility of the "seller," i.e., the *shadchan*, to disclose.

However, if the *shadchan* knows that the family intends to completely withhold this information, this is a serious issue. The *shadchan* should reconsider proposing *shidduchim* for this family.

Preventative Removal of the Ovaries and Sterilization

Q: The removal of the ovaries is often recommended as a preventative measure to reduce the risk of ovarian cancer in women with the BRCA mutation. According to the National Cancer Institute, women with BRCA1 have a 39 percent risk of ovarian cancer, as compared to the 1.4 percent risk of the general population (the percent risk for women with BRCA2 being 11–17 percent). For carriers of high-risk BRCA1 mutations, preventative removal of the ovaries (prophylactic oophorectomy) at around age 40 reduces the risk of ovarian and breast cancer. According to one study, having this surgery at around age 40 increases the woman's chance of reaching age 70 by fifteen percentage points, from 59 percent to 74 percent. However, there is a general halachic issue with destroying reproductive organs. Under what circumstances would halachah allow the removal of the ovaries?

A: We will first clarify whether removing the ovaries or uterus is a Torah or rabbinic prohibition. Next we will analyze if these risks are considered *pikuach nefesh*.

Fundamental Concepts

The Torah clearly forbids destroying the reproductive organs of a male human or animal. The Talmud understands that this prohibition exists even if the organs are presently not functional (termed *me'sareis achar me'sareis*).[273] The Talmud also states that destroying female reproductive organs are prohibited as well, but there is a dispute among later authorities if that prohibition is of Torah or rabbinic origin.[274] Whether the prohibition is a Torah prohibition or rabbinic could impact the level of risk required to consider a situation to be *pikuach nefesh* and therefore override the prohibition.

Rabbi Moshe Feinstein's Discussion

There is a discussion in *Igros Moshe* about a woman undergoing a hysterectomy because her uterus was diseased.[275] Rabbi Moshe Feinstein was asked if the ovaries and fallopian tubes could be removed as well in order to prevent a 5 percent risk of ovarian cancer. He cites the opinion of the Vilna Gaon that castration of the female is a Torah prohibition.[276] He notes that in order to override a Torah prohibition, the risk must be substantial. Nonetheless, Rabbi Feinstein ruled that a one in twenty chance (5 percent) is considered a situation of *pikuach nefesh* — even to override a Torah prohibition.

He also reasons that the prohibition of destroying reproductive organs that are not functional (*me'sareis achar me'sarais*) is limited to male organs, not female. Therefore, in a situation where the woman is infertile or is anyway undergoing a hysterectomy, there is no prohibition of removing additional reproductive organs.

---

273 *Shabbos* 111a; *Shulchan Aruch*, Even HaEzer 5:11–14.

274 See *Otzar HaPoskim*, Even HaEzer 5.

275 Choshen Mishpat 2:73:7.

276 Biur HaGra, Even HaEzer 5:28.

1 in 20

Rabbi Feinstein's assertion that one out of twenty constitutes *pikuach nefesh* is intriguing. The Mishkenos Yaakov, in the laws of kashrus, writes that ten in one-hundred (10 percent) is considered common, while many halachic sources use 1 in 1000 as a definition of something exceedingly rare.[277] There is obviously a huge gap between these numbers. This compels us to consider other factors as well. It is plausible that Rabbi Feinstein's assertion that a 5 percent risk is *pikuach nefesh* is not a definite number. It might only apply to this woman who already has a diseased uterus. This predisposition may establish a *chazakah* that this woman is more vulnerable. However, in a situation where the woman is completely well and the concern is entirely a speculative statistic of 5 percent, it may not be sufficient.[278]

Conclusion

According to many statistics, women with BRCA1 have nearly a forty percent risk of ovarian cancer. This is a very high number compared to the general population, which carries a risk of less than two percent. This is far above the ten percent mentioned by the Mishkenos Yaakov. As such, this clearly establishes this risk as a present and tangible threat, although there are no present signs of illness. Therefore, if there is evidence that a prophylactic oophorectomy significantly lowers the occurrence of cancer, this is considered *pikuach nefesh* and is permitted.

---

277 *Maros HaTzovos*, Even HaEzer 17:98, s.v. *ve'ain zeh*; *Avnei Nezer*, Choshen Mishpat 125.

278 Based on a conversation with Rabbi Dovid Feinstein.

Health Screening and Genetic Testing vs. Bitachon

Q: How do halachic sources view preventative measures like health screenings or genetic testing? Are they included in our obligation to heal or is it a form of speculation that the Torah instructs us not to concern ourselves with?

A: There are a number of very interesting halachic discussions that may be helpful in developing an approach to these types of questions. We will start with the concept of *tomim tihiyeh* — "You shall be wholehearted with Hashem," and develop its implications to our questions.

The Mitzvah of Tomim Tihiyeh

After prohibiting sorcery, the Torah instructs *tomim tihiyeh im Hashem Elokecha* — "You shall be wholehearted with Hashem your G-d."[279] The Sages in the Sifri interpret the verse as warning against conjecturing about the future. The *Shulchan Aruch* rules that "one should not consult star gazers or cast lots [about the future]."[280] The Rema and Shach explain that these practices do not fall under the prohibition of sorcery but are not advisable because of the precept of *tomim tihiyeh*.

Seeking Kabbalists and Fortune-Tellers

In Adar 1987, Rabbi Nosson Gestetner in *Lehoros Nosson* was asked if *tomim tihiyeh* prohibits distraught individuals from seeking purported kabbalists for advice, fortune telling, amulets, palm and face reading, and the like.[281] In response to this question, he wrote a comprehensive

279 *Devarim* 18:13.

280 Yoreh Dei'ah 179:1.

281 6:78–83.

overview of this subject. Rabbi Gestetner points out that according to the Rambam, Terumas HaDeshen, Maharshal, and Shach, *tomim tihiyeh* is not an absolute obligation, though the Torah is urging us to strive to place our faith in Hashem. However, according to the Smag, Ramban, Yerai'im, Smak, and others, it is a concrete obligation and therefore forbidden.

Rabbi Gestetner then makes an important distinction between fortune-telling versus healing with an amulet. When the Rishonim explain this mitzvah, they prohibit gazing into the future and encourage having faith that Hashem determines our destiny. Rabbi Gestetner understands that this prohibition is specific to practices that speculate the future, such as star gazing mentioned in *Shulchan Aruch*. However, healing with an amulet is not an act of telling the future. It is harnessing supernatural powers to heal and bring good fortune. While he questions the authenticity of many of these practices, he writes that they do not violate *tomim tihiyeh* if the objective is not to tell the future.

According to his view, *tomim tihiyeh* is very limited and may not apply to health screenings and genetic testing at all. As he explained, only practices similar to fortune telling are prohibited. Arguably, the results of a health screening or genetic test indicate facts that are in the present, not the future. This is comparable to leaving a glass at the edge of a table. I cannot say that the glass is destined to fall off and break, but its position certainly puts it at greater risk. Likewise, test results showing hypertension or indicating a genetic mutation do not prophesize a future event, rather they indicate a present level of risk. For this reason, health screenings and genetic testing may not be included in the warning of *tomim tihiyeh* because they are quite different from star gazing or psychic readings.

Rabbi Moshe Feinstein on Tomim Tihiyeh

Rabbi Moshe Feinstein took a more expansive understanding of *tomim tihiyeh*. He famously wrote in *Igros Moshe* that it is not necessary for a couple to date excessively to make sure they have found "the right one." He explains: "One should not be overly smart; [rather] the woman who finds favor in his eyes in her appearance and family, and has a good reputation that she is observant, one could rely and marry her with the hope that she is the one destined to him from heaven. He does not need to test her first, and [anyway] it will not help because this testing is nothing, as the verse says *tomim tihiyeh im Hashem* — you shall be wholehearted with Hashem."[282] Rabbi Feinstein is clearly extending the concept of *tomim tihiyeh* to all areas of life, including choosing one's wife. Nonetheless, the implications of this approach needs clarification.

The basis of Rabbi Feinstein's approach is the comments of Rashi on this verse. Rashi explains the mitzvah of *tomim tihiyeh* by saying: "Walk before Hashem with wholeness, hope for Him, and do not speculate about the future. Rather, all that comes upon you accept with wholeness (uncomplicatedness) and then Hashem will be with you." Based on Rashi's comments, Rabbi Feinstein understood that *tomim tihiyeh* is a general instruction to place our faith in Hashem when confronting the unknown.

In 1977, after the Entebbe hijacking and rescue, some yeshivah students wrote to Rabbi Feinstein asking him how this miracle could happen through Jewish soldiers that do not keep the Torah. Rabbi Feinstein dismissed their question by stating simply that we do not understand the ways of Hashem. We should not involve ourselves in these types of analysis, as the verse says *tomim tihiyeh im Hashem*. Here too, Rabbi Feinstein invoked *tomim tihiyeh* as a general instruction to place our faith simply in the hands of Hashem.

Personal Decisions

Although Rabbi Feinstein extolled faith and simplicity, in *Dibros Moshe*, his classic work on the Talmud, he fully acknowledged a person's right to be wise and farsighted about personal matters.[283] The Talmud in *Bava Metzia* states that in certain situations a Torah scholar may say a white lie to avoid embarrassment.[284] Rabbi Feinstein observes that in these scenarios the probability of the embarrassment actually

---

282 1:90.

283 *Bava Metzia* 31:18.

284 23b.

happening is very far-fetched. It does not meet regular halachic standards. He therefore arrived at a fascinating conclusion. The halachic concepts of majority and *chazakah* were only intended as halachic determinations. They are not necessarily a directive when making personal decisions. Therefore, when avoiding embarrassment, which is a personal concern, it is understandable to be concerned even about a minute possibility. Therefore, the Talmud permitted telling a white lie to avoid this eventuality.

Testing for Tay-Sachs

Rabbi Feinstein seems to be balancing these opposing concepts in his discussion about premarital testing for Tay-Sachs. First he writes that since the probability of both spouses being carriers is minute, it may be included in the precept of *tomim tihiyeh*, which according to Rashi instructs us not to delve into the future. However, he then writes that since the test is easily available and an inflicted child is born with devastating disabilities, the public should be educated about their options.[285]

Apparently, there seems to be a relationship between the probability of the occurrence and the severity of the possible outcome. If the risk is not very significant and the outcome is not very damaging, we should rely on faith and not be overly proactive. However, if the outcome is devastating or if the risk is significant, we are encouraged to take the initiative and not rely on faith.

The Maharshal and Maharal on Tomim Tihiyeh

The famed Rabbi Shlomo Luria (1500s) wrote in a responsum that an ill person is not expected to rely on faith alone and may seek a gentile sorcerer or astrologer to heal him.[286] This ruling comes despite the Sages' general disfavor with these unreliable practices. However, Rabbi Luria strongly discourages a well person from such behavior based on *tomim tihiyeh*.

---

285 *Igros Moshe*, Even HaEzer 4:10.

286 *Shu"t Maharshal* #3.

The assertion to differentiate between a sick or well person can be embellished with the comments of the Maharal of Prague in *Nesivos Olam*.[287] The Maharal explains that faith in Hashem is referred to as *temimus* — wholeness, because it is a straight and sensible path. For this reason, seeking astrologers or sorcerers is discouraged because it deviates from a straight and logical approach to life.

With this in mind, we can gain a better appreciation for Rabbi Luria's position. The mitzvah of *tomim tihiyeh* is instructing us to be sensible. Logic dictates that a well person should not be concerned with far-fetched or whimsical possibilities. Instead, he should place his faith in the Master of the World. However, if a person is ill and desperate, it is reasonable that he will seek all possible options, even if they are not reliable.[288] Therefore, under these circumstances it is not a deviation from a straight path.

Cancer Screenings and Routine Checkups

In this light we can understand a conversation of Rabbi Feinstein about cancer screening from the late 1970s.[289] Apparently, a doctor was urging an ostensibly well person to undergo excessive (lit. strange) and possibly dangerous tests. The patient asked Rabbi Feinstein his opinion on the matter. Rabbi Feinstein asserted, based on *tomim tihiyeh*, that if there are no symptoms, there is no reason to seek medical attention. This is because doing so is not part of our normal responsibility to follow *derech hateva* — the natural ways of the world.

It seems that Rabbi Feinstein was concerned with the testing because it was far more excessive than the normative standards of the time. Additionally, the tests carried health risks and were possibly inconclusive. In a similar vein, Rabbi Dovid Feinstein permits pregnant women to go for routine ultrasounds because since it is the common standard of care, it is not an issue of *tomim tihiyeh*.

We can learn from this that the issue of *tomim tihiyeh* only applies

---

287 Nesiv HaTemimus.

288 See Maharal, *Be'er Sheva*, p. 30 (standard edition).

289 *Mesores Moshe*, p. 293.

when the testing is considered excessive compared to standard medical practice. This approach fits very nicely with the teachings of the Maharal that being concerned about unlikely possibilities and excessive testing deviates from a straightforward and sensible approach to life.

With this in mind, we can revisit the issue of routine health checkups:

- If the purpose of the checkup is to check for a rare disease, then *tomim tihiyeh* may view the checkup as superfluous. However, screening for common health problems like hypertension, obesity, high cholesterol, and glucose levels, which could lead to serious health concerns, is quite different. Just as the Rambam encourages us to maintain a healthy lifestyle, regular checkups that focus on keeping our bodies healthy do not conflict with *tomim tihiyeh*.
- Furthermore, as Rabbi Dovid Feinstein noted about ultrasounds, if these practices have become the norm it would not be considered excessive. Therefore it would not be an issue of *tomim tihiyeh*.

Genetic Testing — A Communal Perspective

Contemporary *poskim* discuss the halachic determination of insect infestation in commercial settings like a restaurant or nursing home.[290] The following point could be made: If one insect is commonly found in every crate of lettuce, an individual would not be obligated to check for insects because they only purchase a few heads at a time. However, a caterer may be different. The caterer serving lettuce at an affair uses many heads, and therefore it is likely that one of the guests will eat a bug. Therefore, unlike the private consumer, the caterer would be obligated to check the lettuce.

We can perhaps view the likelihood of genetic diseases in a similar way. About 1 in 30 Ashkenazi Jews are carriers of the Tay-Sachs gene. According to one study, 1 in 3,500 births of Ashkenazi Jews are born with the disease. On one hand, as Rabbi Moshe Feinstein pointed out, the likelihood of a child being born with this dreaded disease is not very high compared to

---

290 See *Emek HaTeshuvah* 8:86; *Minchas Shlomo* 2:63.

other birth defects. However, from a communal perspective with thousands of Jewish children being born each year, one out of 3,500 births is a very real and painful reality that the community must deal with.

Rabbi Elyashiv on Life Insurance

Rabbi Yosef Shalom Elyashiv raised a similar point about buying life insurance. He wrote that it is proper to encourage individuals to buy life insurance because it will ease the communal burden of supporting widows and orphans.[291] Seemingly, Rabbi Elyashiv was addressing the hashkafic argument that buying life insurance demonstrates a lack of trust in Hashem. His response was that if the individual buys the policy because it is in the best interest of the community, it is not an issue. He is not indicating that he is overly concerned that he may die, but is just doing his part to address a legitimate communal problem. While an individual may have the right to say that it is unlikely that he will die prematurely, on a communal level it is a reality that is all too common.

Rabbi Elyashiv's observation about life insurance resonates with our discussion about genetic testing and health screening. In our previous discussions, we addressed these issues from the perspective of the individual. Is it proper to be concerned about getting an unlikely disease or does it conflict with being whole with Hashem? Here we are addressing this question from a different vantage point. If there is significant incidence of these diseases within the community, we are obligated as a community to prevent them through health screenings and genetic testing. As such, the individual's participation is no longer viewed as a lack of *bitachon*; he is instead doing so as part of a community, not out of personal concern.

Summary

- According to Rabbi Nosson Gestetner, the primary obligation of *tomim tihiyeh* is referring to fortune-telling and stargazers, not a medical test that shows a present disposition to a disease.

---

291 *Kovetz Teshuvos* 1:18.

- Rabbi Moshe Feinstein viewed *tomim tihiyeh* as a general directive not to be overly concerned about the future. However, he recognized that when the outcome could be devastating, a person has the right to be concerned about an unlikely possibility.
- According to Rabbi Dovid Feinstein, once a particular test or screening has become commonplace, there is no longer an issue of *tomim tihiyeh*.
- In the teachings of the Maharal of Prague, *tomim tihiyeh* instructs us to be sensible. We should not be overly concerned with far-fetched worries or things that we can't control. However, we should take the logical steps to prevent calamities that can be avoided.
- As Rabbi Elyashiv ruled with life insurance, when an individual does his or her part in preventing a communal tragedy or burden, it does not demonstrate a lack of trust in Hashem.

Anesthesiologist Assisting in an Abortion

Q: A patient wishes to terminate her pregnancy in the second or third trimester. The process requires the assistance of an anesthesiologist to provide either general anesthesia or a regional anesthetic. Is it halachically permissible for a Jewish anesthesiologist to be involved in the care of such a patient — either to initiate or to take over pain management?

A: Although there are varying perspectives about this question, here is a well-balanced approach:

The Concept of Lifnei Iver

The Torah prohibition of facilitating in a transgression, called *lifnei iver*, only applies if one's involvement is crucial in making the transaction happen. If the prohibition will happen anyway, it does not transgress *lifnei iver*. In our question, the patient will still end up aborting the fetus regardless of whether or not the anesthesiologist assists. According to this reasoning, assisting in the abortion would not transgress *lifnei iver*.

However, according to the view of the Mishneh LeMelech, there still may be an issue of *lifnei iver* with abortion.[292] The Mishneh LeMelech maintains that even if the transgression will take place anyway, if *someone* will transgress *lifnei iver*, it is still prohibited to assist. For example, it is not *lifnei iver* to provide nonkosher food to a Jew if he could purchase it from non-Jews. However, if he could only get it from other Jews, according to the Mishneh LeMelech it transgresses *lifnei iver*. This is because *someone* will definitely transgress *lifnei iver* in the process, even if the person will eat it anyway. According to this approach, because the prohibition of abortion applies to Jews and non-Jews, to provide the anesthesia would still be an issue of *lifnei iver*. While many authorities disagree with the Mishneh LeMelech, it would be advisable to avoid such situations if possible. Furthermore, because abortion in many respects is considered murder, there is an extra reason to avoid having any involvement.

Is Administering Anesthesia Considered Aiding in a Transgression?

On the other hand, it can be argued that the anesthesiologist is not really aiding in the abortion at all. The actual abortion is being done by the doctor and the anesthesiologist's role is only in the pain management. Furthermore, the primary role of the anesthesiologist is not during the actual procedure but rather before it. For these reasons, the anesthesiologist's role in facilitating a transgression can be viewed as

---

292 On *Mishneh Torah*, Malveh VeLoveh 4:2.

insignificant. It would seem that in unavoidable situations this reconsideration could be relied upon, especially if it could put the physician's livelihood in jeopardy. Furthermore, if the care had already been initiated, the role of the doctor who is just maintaining it is even more insignificant.[293] Additionally, in many situations, a lethal drug is given to the fetus before the actual D&C. If this is the case, then there is no issue at all because the fetus is no longer living at the time of the D&C.

Embryo Testing for Couple with a Genetic Disease

Q: A husband and wife are carriers of an autosomal recessive trait like Tay-Sachs. Today there is the option of using contraceptives and only having children through in-vitro fertilization. This would allow the embryos to be tested before implantation (PGD) and avoid these devastating diseases. What are the halachic considerations in such a situation?

A: Here is a halachic background on some of the issues involved in this question:[294]

Contraception

The couple will obviously need to use contraceptives in order to prevent any untested pregnancies. While the subject of contraceptives is extensive and sensitive, at this time we will focus on the aspects of this subject pertinent to our question.

---

293 See *Igros Moshe*, Choshen Mishpat 2:73:8; *Shulchan Shlomo*, Refuah 3, p. 108; *Emek HaTeshuvah* 2:93; *Beer Moshe* 5:164.

294 For extensive coverage of these issues, see the contemporary work *Bircas Banim*.

There are two basic halachic concerns with contraceptives: a) neglecting the mitzvah of procreation, which is one of the greatest mitzvos in the Torah; and b) inhibiting conception, which could be considered destroying the male seed (*hash'chasas zera*).

Unlike most questions about contraception, in this situation the couple very much wants to have children. They just want to be spared having a child stricken with a devastating disease. As such, it can be argued that the first concern should not apply, since the couple's intent is to have children.

The next issue that needs to be addressed is the method of contraception. Much of the early halachic discussions about contraception were about using a physical barrier to prevent the sperm from entering the cervix, which both Rabbi Akiva Eiger and the Chasam Sofer ruled is forbidden to do so.[295] However, later authorities maintained that if there is a real danger if the woman becomes pregnant, it is permitted.[296] They reasoned that in this situation, this is considered normal and it is not considered destroying the male seed. Contemporary *poskim* note that the usage of pills and other hormonal therapies do not pose the same issues. These pills inhibit ovulation but the actual path of the sperm does not change. Therefore it is not considered *hash'chasas zera*. However, the Yam Shel Shlomo writes that one should nonetheless not inhibit the normal course of procreation without a pressing reason.[297] Therefore, when making decisions about birth control, rabbinic guidance is always necessary.

Returning to our discussion, there is an important distinction between the method of contraception used. An actual barrier like a diaphragm raises the issue of *hash'chasas zera*. Even according to the more lenient view, it is only permitted if pregnancy could actually put the mother's life in danger, like causing a uterine rupture. In our case, where the pregnancy would not pose a risk to the mother's life, a barrier form of contraception would not be appropriate. Therefore, to avoid

---

295 See *Piskei Teshuvah*, Even HaEzer 23:2.

296 See *Otzar HaPoskim*, Even HaEzer 23.

297 *Yevamos* 6:44, as explained in *Aruch HaShulchan* 5:24.

this issue, a form of contraception that does not create a physical barrier, like hormone pills, should be used. An intrauterine device (IUD) may also be an option.

In Vitro Fertilization

Artificial reproductive technologies have generated much discussion in contemporary rabbinic literature, and there are varying approaches both from a halachic and *hashkafic* standpoint.

Rabbi Moshe Feinstein writes in *Igros Moshe* that if all elements are from the married couple (sperm, ovum, and mother carrying the pregnancy), then in principle artificial reproductive technologies are permitted.[298] However, a primary concern is under what circumstances is it permitted to procure sperm for artificial reproduction (which would normally require *hash'chasas zera*). For example, many *poskim* permit artificial insemination only if the couple did not yet fulfill the mitzvah of procreation.

Our situation is unique. The couple can achieve a pregnancy naturally, but there is a serious possibility of traumatically having a very ill child. A strong argument could be made that sparing themselves this pain is also a legitimate reason. Therefore, this should not be an issue of *hash'chasas zera*. Nonetheless, the method of collection should be as natural as possible.

IVF and the Mitzvah of Procreation (Peru U'Revu)

Q: Does halachah consider a child conceived through in vitro fertilization (IVF) as the child of the biological father? Does he fulfill the mitzvah of *peru u'revu* — procreation?

---

298 Even HaEzer 4:32:5.

A: Long before modern reproductive technologies, the Talmud talks about the concept of artificial reproduction, in specific a case of a woman who conceived by using a warm bath as the conduit for the sperm.[299] Many early commentaries discuss the possible halachic ramifications of this unusual form of conception. Contemporary sources have relied heavily on these discussions when dealing with modern-day questions about artificial reproduction. Here is a short overview of the development and application of these parallels:[300]

- One of the classic commentaries on *Shulchan Aruch*, the Chelkas Mechokek, poses the question if the biological father of a child accidentally conceived through artificial means fulfills *peru u'revu*.
- Another important commentary, the Beis Shmuel, weighs in on this question. He cites Rabbeinu Peretz,[301] a Rishon, who says that a child conceived through artificial means is still considered the son of the biological father. The Beis Shmuel argues that since halachah recognizes the father's paternity, then this should also be a fulfillment of his obligation of procreation.
- Some commentaries (Taz, Maharam Shick)[302] question the Beis Shmuel's reasoning. While the biological father has paternity, how could the mitzvah of procreation be fulfilled accidentally? They contend that paternity and fulfilling the mitzvah are not necessarily linked.
- In modern times, contemporary discussions about artificial insemination and IVF deal with both the question of paternity and the fulfilment of procreation. When considering the question of paternity, many sources see a direct parallel between the comments of Rabbeinu Peretz and today's artificial

299 *Chagigah* 15a.

300 See *Be'er Haitiv*, Even HaEzer 1:9, and *Otzar HaPoskim*.

301 Quoted by the Taz, Yoreh Dei'ah 195:7.

302 Mitzvah 1.

reproductive techniques. Therefore, just as Rabbeinu Peretz still granted paternity to the biological father of a child conceived through unusual means, the same applies to artificial reproductive technologies. Some point out that not all halachic sources necessarily agree with Rabbeinu Peretz.[303] However, Rabbi Moshe Feinstein maintained that since the comments of Rabbeinu Peretz are cited by the Taz, Beis Shmuel, and Mishneh LeMelech without dispute, this is the halachah.[304]

- Does the father fulfill the mitzvah of procreation through artificial reproductive technologies? There is a strong argument that even the Taz and Maharam Shick would agree that artificial reproductive technologies are a fulfilment of this mitzvah. The point of contention between the Beis Shmuel versus the Taz and Maharam Shick was if this mitzvah could be fulfilled accidentally. That would only apply when the father had no intention to father a child. However, in modern times, when a couple seeks infertility treatment, they are consciously trying to fulfill this mitzvah. Therefore, once we accept that halachah recognizes the biological father's paternity, it should follow that he fulfills the mitzvah as well.
- Some contemporary sources take an opposite position on this issue. They feel that the intentional aspect of artificial reproductive technologies actually detracts from the biological father's paternity. They argue that the involvement of the doctor and lab technician facilitating the conception undermines the biological father's connection to the child. This would also impact his fulfillment of procreation as well. However, many contemporary halachic authorities find this notion difficult to accept.[305]

---

303 *Minchas Yitzchak* 1:50.

304 Teshuvos printed in *Dibros Moshe*, Kesubos.

305 *Teshuvos VeHanhagos* 2:690; see *Yabia Omer*, Even HaEzer 2:1 for a comprehensive overview of contemporary sources on this subject.

Abortion and Fetal Anomalies

Q: Is it permissible for a Jewish person to have an abortion for fetal anomalies, and if so, under what circumstances? Does it matter how far along it is in the pregnancy (forty days, etc.)?

A: The question of abortion in these situations is a sensitive one and requires direction from an expert *posek* — halachic authority. On one hand, there is the priceless value of human life. On the other hand, there is the emotional anguish of the couple. Let us consider a brief overview of the halachic literature on this subject.

Classic Sources

The Rambam writes that if during labor the mother's life is in danger because of the fetus, the mother's life takes precedence. This is because the fetus has the status of a *rodef* — a pursuer, who the Torah permits killing to save the pursued.

The Nodah BeYehudah, Maharam Shick, Rabbi Chaim Soloveitchik, Rabbi Moshe Feinstein, and Rogochover Gaon all focus on why the Rambam needed to label the unborn fetus a *rodef* to permit aborting it. They conclude that the prohibition of abortion is murder, one of the three cardinal sins, and the normal rules of *pikuach nefesh* do not apply. Therefore, the danger to the mother's life alone would not be a sufficient reason to permit aborting the fetus. The Rambam only permitted aborting the fetus because it has the status of a *rodef* whose life may be terminated in order to save the pursued.[306]

However, the Toras Chesed of Lublin understands that the stringent position of the Rambam on abortion is only applicable when the

306 *Yabia Omer*, Even HaEzer 4:1, citing *Nodah BeYehudah* and Rogochover Gaon, *Chidushei R' Chaim HaLevi* on Rambam; *Igros Moshe*, Choshen Mishpat 2:69–71.

woman is in active labor.[307] At that point, the fetus is no longer a part of her body and is already considered its own life. However, during the pregnancy, the fetus is just considered a part of the mother's body and does not have this status. According to this approach, an early abortion is still a Torah prohibition (like keeping Shabbos or eating kosher) but is not one of the three cardinal sins. This means that in certain situations there would be more room for leniency than according to the first approach. Rabbi Chaim Ozer Grodzensky of pre-WWII Vilna concurs with this approach.[308]

Another point of contention is the position of Tosfos on abortion. Tosfos seems to hold that abortion is permitted for maternal considerations, even if the concern is not life-threatening. The problem is that even according to this approach, abortion would still be considered murder for non-Jews.[309] It is ironic that abortion could be more permissive for Jews than non-Jews. Nonetheless, the Sheilas Yaavetz and Chavos Yair take such an approach. The Maharit possibly agreed with this as well.

Contemporary Views

In 1975, Rabbi Eliezer Yehudah Waldenberg was asked by Shaare Zedek hospital if abortion could be permitted for a couple carrying a fetus with Tay-Sachs disease. After considering the seriousness of the issue, Rabbi Waldenberg writes that abortion could be permitted until the seventh month of pregnancy. This ruling was based on his understanding of Tosfos, the Maharit, Yaavetz, and Chavos Yair.[310]

Rabbi Moshe Feinstein sharply criticized Rabbi Waldenberg's position. He questioned the reliability of Tosfos's comments. He pointed out that the Maharit's lenient responsum seems to be contradicted by another responsum a few chapters later.[311] Rabbi Shlomo Zalman Auerbach is quoted in *Nishmas Avraham* as leaning to be stringent like

307 2:42–44.

308 *Achiezer* 3:72.

309 See *Sanhedrin* 57b; *Mishneh Torah*, Melachim 9:4.

310 *Tzitz Eliezer* 13:102; *Emek HaTeshuvah* 2:92 takes a similar position.

311 *Igros Moshe*, Choshen Mishpat 2:69–71.

Rabbi Feinstein.[312] Additionally, the halachic responsa of Rabbi Ovadia Yosef, Rabbi Shmuel Wosner, and Rabbi Yosef Shalom Elyashiv do not seem to accept Rabbi Waldenberg's permissive ruling regarding Tay-Sachs.

Forty Days

The Talmud famously writes that until forty days from conception, the fetus is "like water."[313] The Beis Shlomo and other sources understand that before forty days, the prohibition of abortion is not as strict.[314] Based on this consideration, Rabbi Yechiel Yaakov Weinberg in *Sridai Aish* permitted an English doctor to perform an abortion of a fetus infected with German measles before forty days.[315] However, Rabbi Feinstein disagreed with this approach.[316] He maintained that from the fact that Shabbos is desecrated to save a fetus before forty days, it must still be considered a life. He infers that a fetus may not be aborted even at this early stage.

Fetal Anomalies

Rabbi Shmuel Wosner in *Shevet HaLevi* discusses situations where the fetus has serious abnormalities in the brain or heart and cannot live very long after birth. He leans toward the approach of the Toras Chesed, who views abortion as a Torah prohibition but not one of the three cardinal sins. Moreover, he argues that if unfortunately the fetus is a *treifah* that cannot survive for twelve months or a *nefel* that cannot live for thirty days, its status is further compromised. Therefore, in a situation where the mother is in great anguish, one could permit aborting the fetus (although it is after forty days).[317] However, it does not seem that the first group of opinions would necessarily agree with this approach.

---

312 *Nishmas Avraham*, Choshen Mishpat 425.

313 *Yevamos* 69b.

314 Choshen Mishpat 132.

315 *Sridai Aish*, Choshen Mishpat 162.

316 See *Igros Moshe*, Choshen Mishpat 2:69.

317 *Shevet HaLevi* 9:266.

Mental Health Complications

We have mentioned that if a mother's life is in danger during labor, the fetus may be aborted. There is an interesting question if this is limited to physical complications or it even applies to psychiatric issues. The Levushai Mordechai considered serious psychiatric issues resulting from the pregnancy as legitimate maternal considerations. Likewise, Rabbi Feinstein viewed the risk of a nervous breakdown as a legitimate reason to abort although it is not directly caused by the fetus.[318]

Summary[319]

- Rabbi Feinstein only permitted aborting a fetus when there is a real risk of life to the mother. He did not differentiate between stages of pregnancy.
- If the fetus has a lethal condition and can only live for a few days after birth, some permit abortion as long as the fetus is completely dependent on the mother.
- If the condition is not lethal but a serious disorder like Tay-Sachs, some permit aborting before forty days but not after.
- Rabbi Waldenberg permitted aborting a fetus with Tay-Sachs even after forty days, but many of his contemporaries did not agree with him.

---

318 *Reshumai Aharon* [Felder], Choshen Mishpat 425:4.

319 See Dr. A. Steinberg's *Encyclopedia of Medical Halachah* for further sources.

Helping a Patient Choose Which Rabbi to Ask

Q: A Jewish patient is trying to decide who to ask her halachic question to and asks which rabbinic authority (*posek*) might permit an abortion in her situation. Is it appropriate to tell her the name of a *posek* who the doctor knows has permitted abortions in similar situations?

A: This important question touches on many issues, including the entire concept of the halachic decision-making process. Let's summarize the relevant concepts:

Methodology of Halachic Decision Making

The Rema gives direction to how a rabbi should render a halachic decision when there are differing opinions:[320]

- If the rabbi is a great scholar, he can prove which opinion seems more correct;
- If not, he can use the general rule of doubt — to be stringent with Torah prohibitions and lenient with rabbinic prohibitions;
- Or follow the majority opinion;
- Or follow a prevailing custom to rely on the ruling of a particular scholar that became accepted in that place, even if it is a minority opinion.[321]

Following a Minority Opinion in Extenuating Circumstances

As the Rema mentioned, when there is a difference of opinion, we

---

320 Choshen Mishpat 25:2.

321 Interestingly, the Pri Chadash explains that the Sephardic customs generally follow the rulings of the Rambam, whereas the Ashkenazic customs usually follow the opinions of the Rosh and Tosfos, because these were the leading halachic authorities in their lands, and by accepting them as their teachers they became bound to them.

generally follow the majority. However, the Talmud writes that if the halachah has not clearly been decided, the great scholar of the Mishnah, Rabbi Shimon Bar Yochai, can be relied upon in a situation of great need, even though his opinion is a minority view. Based on this, the Shach and Taz both write that an important opinion in a case of great necessity can sometimes be relied upon.[322] However, they disagree how far reaching this concept can be taken. The Shach maintains that it only applies to a rabbinic prohibition, while the Taz seems to allow relying on a minority opinion in extenuating circumstances even with Torah prohibitions. This opinion of the Taz is very puzzling, for wouldn't following a minority opinion contradict the biblical command to follow the majority?

The comments of the Tashbatz shed some light onto this issue. He writes that this rule depends on a number of factors: whether the question at hand is of Torah or rabbinic origin, whether it is an earlier dispute where a clear consensus has already been reached or a more contemporary question where the lines have not been clearly drawn, and whether the minority opinion is shared by others or if it is entirely the opinion of a single individual.[323] Based on the Tashbatz, we can explain why this concept does not necessarily contradict the idea of following the majority. The full obligation to follow the majority is when there is a clear consensus. However, if the question is more contemporary, or if there is not an overwhelming majority, there is room for leniency in extenuating circumstances.

Asking a Shailah

The Talmud writes that until there was a final consensus to accept the ruling of the school of Hillel over the school of Shamai, a person could choose which school he wished to belong to. The Chazon Ish understands this to be a general rule — that a person can choose to follow the opinions of a specific rabbi if he is consistent with his opinion in most areas of halachah, even if it is not a majority opinion.[324]

Rabbi Moshe Feinstein in *Dibros Moshe* adds another dimension to

---

322 Taz, Yoreh Dei'ah 307:(4); Nekudos HaKesef; see *Yabia Omer* 8, Orach Chaim 34:6 for extensive sources on this subject.

323 Cited in *Yabia Omer* ibid.

324 *Chazon Ish*, Yoreh Dei'ah 150:1.

this topic.[325] The Talmud relates that Rabbah Bar Chuna ate a certain fat that other rabbis deemed to be forbidden. Rabbah Bar Chuna explained that he is permitted to eat it because he heard the ruling from the mouth of Rebbe Yochanan, but that others may not [eat it] because it is a minority opinion.[326] Rabbi Feinstein understands from this vignette an important dimension to the halachic decision-making process: hearing a ruling from the mouth of its originator gives the inquirer the right to rely on it regardless of whether or not others agree. Rabbi Feinstein points out however that this is only true if it is heard from the great sage who came up with the ruling or possibly a disciple — certainly not from a disciple's student. This therefore seems to be the underlying principle in asking a halachic question. By asking the question, the inquirer has the right to rely on the opinion of that rabbi, even if others disagree.

Rabbi Feinstein's approach gives important direction when posing a halachic query in a serious situation. The inquirer may ask a rabbi who may rule more leniently, even if others disagree. However, as Rabbi Feinstein explained, that rabbi must be the originator of the ruling or at least his disciple. This means that the rabbi needs to be of the stature that he can defend his position on the issue.

Advising Others

Advising others obviously complicates matters. There is discussion in halachic literature about the balance between the obligation to help others in need (derived from the obligation to return a lost object), and not impeding the judicial process[327] — as the Sages said: "Do not act as a legal advisor."[328]

In our situation, helping the patient find the right rabbi who has the time, patience, sensitivities, halachic expertise, and medical understanding is clearly helping the halachic process and is a great mitzvah. The more difficult question is, when the practitioner, based on previous experience, has a feel how certain rabbis may rule in this situation and

325 *Shabbos* 10.

326 *Pesachim* 51a.

327 See *Seder HaDin*, ch. 16.

328 *Avos* 1:8.

could direct the patient to the rabbi that will give the answer "they want."[329]

As mentioned before, in a *sha'as hadchak* — a situation of great need, it may be permitted to follow a minority opinion. In addition, according to the *Dibros Moshe*, a person may follow the ruling of a great rabbi if he heard the ruling directly from him.[330] However the concept of *sha'as hadchak* is very subjective and it needs to be the inquirer's personal choice to rely on the minority opinion, not that of the advisor.

Conclusion

The decision to rely or consult a minority opinion must come from the patient. Therefore the role of the counselor is to provide accurate and balanced information. As such, if in that particular situation most rabbis would not permit an abortion but some would, the patient should be made aware of exactly this. If with the proper information the patient chooses to take a more lenient approach, he should be directed to consult a rabbi of stature who can defend his position on the matter, as stipulated in the *Dibros Moshe*.

A final thought: often medical practitioners unavoidably become involved in the halachic decision-making process. However, if the patient has a spiritual leader who can responsibly direct them to the halachic authority he should consult, this could alleviate the medical practitioner's burden of giving advice in an area that may be outside his expertise.

---

329 This issue could be compared to the rabbinic prohibition of *ha'arama*, circumventing a prohibition, although the guidelines of when it does or does not apply are unclear.

330 According to the Shoel U'Mashiv and Maharsham (1:81, 82), a *ha'arama* can possibly be permitted in a *sha'as hadchak*.

Aborting a Fetus with Anencephaly

Q: A woman is pregnant with an anencephalic fetus at twenty weeks. Is it permitted to perform an abortion, given the universal adverse outcome for the fetus?

[**Anencephaly** is the absence of a major portion of the brain and skull that occurs during embryonic development. It is accepted that children born with this disorder usually only lack the large upper brain including the neocortex that is responsible for cognition. With very few exceptions, infants with this disorder do not survive longer than a few hours or possibly days after their birth.]

A: This is a unique question. Does the fact that the fetus's brain is so compromised and that the prognosis is so poor impact its status in halachah? According to Rabbi Moshe Feinstein in *Igros Moshe*, an unborn fetus is already viewed as a full life.[331] Based on this approach the poor prognosis of the fetus after birth should not change its present status. Therefore, an abortion could only be permitted if the deterioration of the brain is enough to consider it to be already "dead" at this time. As we have mentioned, anencephaly primarily affects the upper brain but the brain stem remains intact, and since the heart is beating and there is brain stem function, the fetus is far from being "dead." This is comparable to a person who is in a coma after suffering severe injury to the upper brain but their brain stem is intact. Although he may never regain consciousness, he is obviously still viewed as living. As such, unless there is a danger to the life of the mother, it would be forbidden to abort the fetus.[332]

However, Rabbi Shmuel Wosner in *Shevet HaLevi* makes an interesting argument. He understands that the prohibition of aborting a fetus is based on its potential to become a viable human being. As such, since

331 Choshen Mishpat, 2:69–70.

332 In personal communication with Rabbi Dovid Feinstein.

this fetus could only survive for a short period of time after birth, it has a different halachic status. It is comparable to a *nefel* — a fetus unable to live for thirty days, although it is still living. Therefore, there may not be the full prohibition of murder on such a form of life. Based on this logic and other considerations, Rabbi Wosner writes that if the mother is in great distress, there is room for leniency.[333] From a different angle, Rabbi Yitzchok Zilberstein writes that there may be a Talmudic source to consider this form of brain damage severe enough to detract from a fetus's status as a life.[334]

Halachic Considerations for Genetic Counselors

Q: What are the halachic considerations with the practice of genetic counseling?

[Genetic counselors help families and individuals understand and adjust to a heredity diagnosis or disorder and address psychological and ethical issues, which includes aiding patients in making an informed choice about aborting a fetus with genetic problems.]

A: It is important to understand a number of pertinent halachic principles in order to develop an approach to the practice of genetic counseling that is both halachically appropriate and professional.

Providing Information vs. Making a Decision

Although human beings have free will, we are responsible to direct a person toward a specific decision. The Mabit, an important early

333 *Shevet HaLevi* 7:208, 9:266.

334 *Shiurim LeRofim* 4:239. See, however, *Lehoros Nosson* (5:114), who disagrees with Rabbi Zilberstein on this point.

Acharon, held a person liable for convincing some wealthy donors to leave a shul, which caused indirect damages.[335] Apparently then, we are responsible for influencing people's decisions even though they are free to choose what they want. Likewise, Rabbi Moshe Feinstein writes that hosting an event on Shabbos that will cause people to drive to it, may carry a rabbinic prohibition of *masis* — persuading a person to do a transgression.[336] However, Rabbi Zilberstein suggests that providing such information in a nondirective way avoids these issues.[337]

According to the secular ethical principle of patient autonomy, the patient is encouraged to make his own decision. The counselor's role is primarily to provide information and understanding. Using a nondirective approach is much less problematic than directing a person toward a specific decision. The counselor is leaving the decision up to the patient and is therefore not responsible for it.

Another point to consider is that when showing empathy and understanding for the patient's decision, the counselor should avoid supporting the correctness of the decision. Rather the focus should be on supporting them emotionally. This approach could avoid the issue of *chanifah* — condoning improper conduct.

Causing or Aiding in a Transgression

Is explaining the unfortunate facts of a situation considered causing or aiding in a transgression if it may lead the parents to decide to have an abortion? The basic principle of *lifnei iver*, the Torah prohibition to cause others to sin, is exclusively when the transgression will only take place with your involvement. Therefore, although providing information may help them decide to terminate the pregnancy, the truth is that the outcome probably would have happened anyway. Even without this specific genetic counselor's involvement, they would have been assigned to a different counselor who would have provided similar information. Furthermore, today the basic information is readily available in many

---

335 3:48.

336 *Igros Moshe*, Orach Chaim 1:99.

337 *Shiurim LeRofim* 4:273.

other forms as well. Therefore it is difficult to contend that the counselor is directly causing a person to transgress the Torah.

In a similar vein, Rabbi Naftali Tzvi Yehudah Berlin, the dean of the Volozhin Yeshivah, was asked if it is permitted to make marriage matches between nonobservant Jewish men and women. The issue is that they will most probably not keep the laws of Jewish family purity, which may be *lifnei iver*. The Netziv, however, did not consider this to be *lifnei iver* because the person may marry even without this involvement.[338] As we have learned, there is only a prohibition of *lifnei iver* if the transgression can only happen with your involvement.

In addition to the Torah prohibition of *lifnei iver*, there is a rabbinic prohibition of *misayeia*. The Sages restricted us from aiding in a transgression even if it will happen anyway. This is because lending aid, even when the transgression is inevitable, is the antithesis of being concerned that a Jew should not sin. However, many opinions maintain that if the involvement is not at the time of the prohibition, it is not included in the restriction of *misayeia*. That approach would definitely apply to a genetic counselor. Counseling usually does not take place at the actual time of the transgression, but in advance. Therefore, according to these opinions it would not be an issue of *misayeia*. However, the Netziv writes that some Rishonim maintain that this leniency only applies when there is a legitimate reason to explain why a person is engaging in this behavior, like financial gain or *darkei shalom* — maintaining peaceful relationships with our neighbors. Nonetheless, in the setting of genetic counseling, there are usually both reasons: firstly it could be an issue of *darkei shalom* in avoiding animosity, as well as a financial interest.

Preventing a More Severe Offense

Rabbi Moshe Feinstein and Rabbi Shlomo Zalman Auerbach discuss situations of *misayeia* in which the transgression is going to happen anyway, but where lending aid could actually prevent a more severe offense. They both understand that the aid can actually be viewed as

338 *Mashiv Davar* 2:32.

preventing a transgression and not aiding in one, which would therefore be permitted.[339]

Likewise, there is a strong argument that having counselors who are sensitive to the value of human life can make the difference in avoiding unnecessary abortions. They can help couples explore other options and support their moral convictions. As such, the practice of genetic counseling can be viewed in general as *afrushai me'isurah* — helping avoid transgression. As such, their unavoidable involvement in cases where a prohibited abortion is taking place could be justified.

Other Mitigating Factors

There are two other mitigating factors to be considered when addressing the concerns of facilitating and aiding in a transgression:

According to Tosfos in *Avodah Zara*, there is no prohibition of *lifnei iver* if the transgression is being done by a third party (*lifnei de'lifnei*).[340] Therefore, the Rema writes that a Jew may sell animals through a non-Jewish broker, even though the customer will castrate them, because the castration is being done by a third party.[341] The Terumas HaDeshen understands that this is so even if the transgression is certain. This concept should apply to genetic counseling as well. The patient coming to the genetic counselor to discuss a termination is not the one primarily doing the transgression, rather the doctor (although the patient is aiding somewhat). Arguably, the prohibition is being done by a third party and is not a Torah violation of *lifnei iver*.

Furthermore, the Noahide prohibition of abortion may be less severe if the fetus has a lethal condition. The Rambam writes that a non-Jew is even prohibited to murder a fetus, or a *treifah* — someone terminally ill, or to cause death indirectly. Some understand that the value of a fetus's life is because it has the potential to become a full human being. Likewise, the Talmud explains that it is prohibited to hasten the death of a *goseis* because he has a *chezkas chiyus* — a pre-existing status

339 See *Igros Moshe*, Yoreh Dei'ah 1:72, s.v. *al kol panim*; *Minchas Shlomo* vol 1, 35:1.

340 15b, s.v. *le'ovaid kochavim*.

341 Even HaEzer 5.

as a viable human being. Therefore, even in the final stages of illness, hastening death is considered murder. According to this approach, it is plausible that a fetus with a lethal condition is different than a *treifah*. The fetus had no pre-existing status as living, and unfortunately does not have the potential to become a viable human being. Therefore, this may not carry the full severity of murder mentioned by the Rambam.[342]

Likewise, there may be difference in the prohibition of euthanasia between a Jew and non-Jew. Although a Jewish person is prohibited to perform euthanasia, Rabbi Moshe Sternbuch postulates that a non-Jew does not have this prohibition.[343] He suggests that because the intent is not to harm but to have mercy, it is not included in the Noahide prohibition of murder. While not all sources point to this approach, Rabbi Y. Zilberstein cites the Yad Ramah on *Bava Basra*,[344] which seems to support this notion.[345] As such, it is possible that a non-Jew who aborts a fetus in order to spare it the pain of its degenerative condition may not be liable for murder.[346]

Summary

The practice of genetic counseling by individuals with a fundamental value for human life, as well as a respect for the halachic process, is of great value to the Jewish community. When dealing with patients who may not share the same values, the observant counselor should avoid a directive approach. Instead, he should show empathy for the difficulty of the situation and provide accurate information so the family can reach its own decision. The halachic concerns are more substantial in cases like Down's syndrome, where the fetus does not have a lethal condition and would not suffer from a painful degenerative disease.

342 See *Teshuvos VeHanhagos* 3:365; *Emek HaTeshuvah* 2:90.

343 *Teshuvos VeHanhagos* ibid.

344 16a.

345 *Shiurim LeRofim* 4:286.

346 Ibid.

Ambiguous Genitalia in Halachah

Q: A baby was born whose chromosome tests determine it to be female, and scans reveal hidden ovaries and a uterus. Externally, however, the clitoris is enlarged and looks like a male organ with some foreskin, but the urethra does not pass through it, and the doctors explain that this problem is caused by an enzyme deficiency in breaking down the testosterone into estrogen. The doctors would like to do hormonal therapy that would help the uterus and ovaries develop and ultimately perform a minor surgery to open the vaginal septum and remove the male organ, which should result in this individual becoming a fertile female. Being that externally the baby looks male, and chromosome tests are a discovery of modern times, how does halachah view this situation? Is this possibly the androgynous (hermaphrodite) mentioned often in Mishnah and Talmud?

A: This question is most fascinating but at the same time very serious and possibly tragic. If we consider this child a male, although scientifically it is female, the child will not be able to marry as a woman and will be stuck in limbo. Thankfully, although this occurrence is not common, it has been responsibly dealt with in both classic and contemporary halachic literature.[347] Here is an overview — with a twist of my own:

Classic and Contemporary Sources

- In 1971, Dr. Shustheim asked Rabbi Waldenberg of Shaare Zedek hospital about a baby who externally had no male organs

347 See the contemporary work *Dor Tahapuchos* and The Encyclopedia of Jewish Medical Ethics for extensive sources.

and looked female, but tested as male.[348] The doctors felt that it would be easier to make the baby into a female,[349] but they were faced with the problem that if halachah would go according to the chromosome test, then this child would not be able to marry a man. Rabbi Waldenberg responded that halachically gender is determined based on the presence of organs and therefore if there are no apparent external male organs, the child can be considered female. Based on Rabbi Waldenberg's approach, it would seem that in our situation where the appearance is male, we would have to consider the child as such. However, after careful study, it does not seem to be the case.

- About two hundred years ago, the Shailas Yaavetz described a situation very similar to ours. An infant had an enlarged clitoris with foreskin, however the urethra was completely open and urinated from the base like a female. The author of the work *Kineses Yechezkel*, a leading rabbi at the time, was asked if there is a mitzvah of circumcision and he responded that there was. Rabbi Yaakov Emden sharply criticized this approach, saying that since the male organ is not functional, it is not halachically considered a male organ, "just flesh." Therefore, the child is a female and we do not circumcise females![350] Based on Rabbi Emden's argument, because in our situation the male organ is not functional, it would not make the child into a male.
- The Talmud often speaks of an androgynous (hermaphrodite). According to the Rambam, it has both male and female reproductive organs. Since the question of what is its halachic status is unresolved, we must be stringent in all respects, and therefore it can only marry a female but must keep mitzvos like a male etc.[351] According to Rabbi Asher Weiss, a contemporary halachic authority, in order to be in this state of limbo, the

---

348 *Tzitz Eliezer* 11:78.

349 Rabbi Waldenberg's discussion was from the early 1970s. However, current medical opinion is against this practice, because emotionally and psychologically the child is the opposite gender.

350 #171.

351 *Mishneh Torah*, Ishus 2:24.

individual must possess a complete set of both male and female organs, i.e., a true hermaphrodite, which is very rare in humans, not a pseudo-hermaphrodite, which is the more common case. According to this approach, even if we would consider this child to possess one male organ, due to the fact that there are no testicles, it would not have the status of an androgynous. It could be more comparable to the case of a *tumtum*, where the genitals are covered and the scans revealing uterus and ovaries would determine the gender of the child. An early responsa of the Rama Mipano may support this approach.

- Rabbi Shmuel Wosner discusses a case like ours and concludes that the child can be considered female because there are no testicles, which are the principle male organ, but there are ovaries and a uterus, the principle female organs. Although the uterus and ovaries are not externally visible, Rabbi Wosner writes that because they could be viewed surgically, that is enough to determine the child's gender.[352]

A Novel Approach

Here is a thought of my own: The Magen Avraham understands the case of androgynous in a peculiar way, explaining that it switches from being male or female from one month to the next (!).[353] (The commentary Machtzis HaShekel asks on the Magen Avraham why this person is not considered each respective gender when it is in that state.) Other commentaries, though, dismiss the approach of the Magen Avraham. Similarly, Rabbi Chaim Palagi, known for discussing all sorts of hypothetical situations, writes that a married woman who miraculously becomes male does not need to be divorced! This is because she is no longer a woman and there is no concept of marriage between two males. From these sources, it seems that gender is determined by a person's present state, not how they were born.

Based on this, we make an interesting argument. The Tzitz Eliezer

---

352 *Shevet HaLevi* 6:149.

353 589:2.

understood that gender is determined according to what is visible externally, not what is shown in the laboratory or even what comes as a result of surgery. Therefore if a child looks male, even if it tests female, then he is male. However, we have learned that gender could change and is based on the present state of being. As such, once this child receives hormonal therapy and the internal organs become palpable, it will then be considered female.

This phenomenon can be explained further. The argument of the Tzitz Eliezer is apparently based on the approach found in many areas of halachah that halachah only works with what the eye can see. That is why microscopic insects are not a problem to eat and microscopic scales on a fish will not make it kosher. In earlier generations, they kept the Torah without these instruments. Likewise, chromosomes, or possibly impalpable internal organs, may not determine gender. However, once the hormones make the internal organs palpable, and especially once the vaginal septum is opened, even in the times of Chazal this individual would definitely have been considered female. If so, then just as the Machtzis HaShekel and Rabbi Chaim Palagi only view the present status, even if this child had the status of androgynous at birth, it would be considered female after the hormones.

Incubator in Halachah (Pidyon Haben, Aveilus)

Q: A preterm infant spent a few months in an incubator. How does halachah view this time regarding *pidyon haben*? Does the thirty-day waiting period required before performing a *pidyon haben* begin from when the baby was born or from when it left the incubator? Similarly, in the laws of mourning, shivah is only observed if an infant lived for thirty days. If a child was in an incubator for thirty days before passing away, does the family observe shivah?

A: In both the laws of redeeming the first-born and the laws of mourning, a child must live for thirty days to create an obligation of *pidyon haben* or shivah. Until thirty days from birth, halachah views the child as possibly a *nefel* — a fetus that is not viable. A *nefel* does not have the full status of a human being in many areas of halachah. As such, an infant who spent much of its first thirty days in an incubator raises an interesting question. Can the time spent in the incubator be counted toward the thirty days needed to remove the concern of *nefel*, or does the child's dependence on the incubator detract from counting these days?

Early Rabbinic Discussions about Incubators

One of the earlier discussions of this question was between Rabbi Akiva Sofer,[354] the last *rav* of Pressburg and descendant of the Chasam Sofer, and Rabbi Mordechai Leib Winkler, author of the *Levushai Mordechai*.[355] Rabbi Sofer maintained that the child is not considered a *nefel* even though it needs the incubator to survive. He compared it to a case in the Talmud in *Chulin* where an artificial covering was made for an

---

354 *Da'as Sofer*, Yoreh Dei'ah 114.

355 *Levushai Mordechai* 3, Orach Chaim 14:2.

animal that had a hole in its windpipe. Though an animal with a hole in its windpipe is a *treifah* and not kosher, the Talmud held that the artificial covering is sufficient to deem the animal not a *treifah*. Rabbi Sofer points out that although the animal needs the artificial covering to survive, once it has it, the animal is no longer considered a *treifah*. In the same way, an infant who is only able to survive in the artificial conditions of the incubator should not be considered a *nefel*. Just like the case in *Chulin*, as long as it is viable with this intervention, this is sufficient.

Rabbi Winkler, in his response to Rabbi Sofer, questioned the comparison between the viability of an infant to the laws of *treifos*. The halachic definition of a *treifah* is a person or animal that has a condition (like a hole in a major organ) that will cause it to die within twelve months. However, a *nefel* is a fetus that never reached the halachic threshold of being fully alive. There is a big difference between being almost alive or almost dead! It is possible that the Talmud only accepted an artificial intervention with a *treifah* in order to maintain its status of being alive. However, it may not be sufficient to give a fetus the initial status of a full human being.

Contemporary Discussions

Since the days of Rabbi Sofer and Rabbi Winkler, there has been much discussion about incubators in the laws of *pidyon haben* and *aveilus*. The focal point of these discussions seems to be how to view the incubator. Everyone would agree that if a newborn needs medicine to survive, the child is still considered "born" and the thirty days begin immediately from birth. In the same way, many *poskim* view the incubator as only playing a supportive role and therefore no different than medicine. Therefore they consider the child to be "born" even though it needs the incubator to live. Others argue that an incubator plays a much more central role than medicine. It is a simulation of being inside the mother. Therefore as long as the child needs the incubator to survive, it still is not considered halachically "born," and the thirty days do not begin until it leaves the incubator and can function independently.

A number of contemporary sources do not obligate the observance of shivah for an infant that did not live for thirty days outside the incubator.[356] This should indicate that the consensus is to view a child in an incubator as unborn. However, this approach does not seem to carry over to *pidyon haben*. Rabbi Moshe Sternbuch writes in *Teshuvos VeHanhagos* that common practice is to perform a *pidyon haben* once thirty days has passed since the birth itself, regardless of whether the child was in an incubator.[357] This approach seems to view the child in the incubator as born, the opposite of the consensus in the laws of mourning.

Explaining the Common Practice

There may be good reason for this dichotomy. The obligation to sit shivah is rabbinic and is governed by the principle that we follow the more lenient opinion in the laws of *aveilus*.[358] This is the reason shivah is not observed on an infant less than thirty days old since we are not sure if it had the status of a *nefel*, and based on the general rule we are lenient when in doubt. Likewise, contemporary *poskim* do not necessarily view the child in the incubator as unborn. Rather, being completely dependent on the incubator at least creates a doubt whether the child is a *nefel* even after thirty days. As such, following the general rule of leniency in the laws of mourning, the family cannot be obligated to observe shivah.

On the other hand, the thirty days of *pidyon haben* is actually a Torah decree. For this reason, a *pidyon haben* is done after thirty days even if the child is full term and completely healthy. As such, the argument not to count the time spent in the incubator is weaker. While an infant dependent on an incubator may not be viable, it is not unborn. Therefore, because the thirty days of *pidyon haben* is not connected to viability, but is a Torah decree, it is logical to count the thirty days from birth. Nonetheless, a *pidyon haben* should not be done if the child may have the status of a *nefel*. As such, Rav Sternbuch suggests that they should wait to perform the *pidyon haben* until the baby leaves the incubator and is self-sufficient, albeit not for thirty days.

---

356 *Shevet HaLevi* 3:143; *Emek HaTeshuvah* 2:90; *Minchas Shlomo* 2:96:5;, see *Yabia Omer* 9, Yoreh Dei'ah 37 for extensive sources.

357 *Teshuvos VeHanhagos* 3:330.

358 "*Halachah kidiveri hameikil be'aveilus.*"

SECTION VI:

END OF LIFE AND TRANSPLANTS

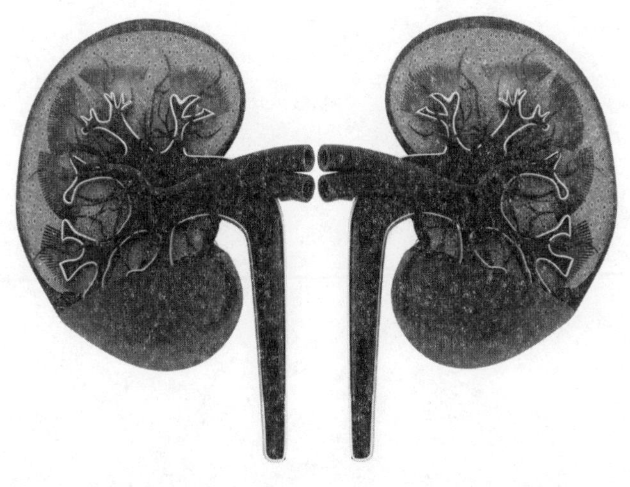

Moving a Goseis (Patient near Death)

Q: Here are two important questions about the prohibition to move a *goseis*, a dying patient:

- Is it permitted to move a *goseis* to facilitate the care of other patients?
- Often, a patient who is possibly a *goseis* becomes soiled. In order to be cleaned the patient needs to be moved. How do we balance *kavod habrios* — human dignity, with the prohibition of moving a *goseis*?

A: We will first consider if a *goseis* may be moved to facilitate the care of other patients. Rabbi Shmuel Wosner makes some very interesting points on this topic:[359]

Defining the Prohibition to Move a Goseis

- The Talmud writes that touching or moving a *goseis* is akin to bloodshed because these actions may hasten its death.[360] It is interesting that the Talmud only refers to direct contact with the patient. Rabbi Wosner reasons that it is possible that indirect contact, like wheeling the bed, may not be included in this concern. Such forms of indirect contact may be too subtle to be of concern.
- The Talmud also writes that if a building collapses on Shabbos,

359 *Shevet HaLevi* 9:245.

360 *Shabbos* 151a.

the rubble and bodies should be removed immediately in order to save any live people trapped underneath.[361] Rabbi Wosner raises an interesting point. If moving a *goseis* is like bloodshed, why does the Talmud imply that in all circumstances the victims should be removed to help find people underneath; perhaps one of the victims is a *goseis* and should not be moved? It seems that although the Talmud writes that moving a *goseis* is akin to bloodshed, it is only a concern that it may hasten death, not a definite risk. Therefore, in situations where there is a more concrete risk at hand, like saving people buried alive in the rubble, that takes precedence over the general concern of moving a *goseis*.

- Furthermore, Rabbi Wosner points out that the exact definition of when a patient has the status of a *goseis* is unclear.

For these reasons, if there is a need to touch or move the patient to facilitate the patient's care or the care of others, it may be done with extreme care. There is particular reason to be lenient if the contact is indirect, such as wheeling a bed.

Human Dignity vs. Moving a Goseis

We will now consider if it is permitted to move a patient who may be a *goseis* to be cleaned. Here are a few points to consider:

- The term *goseis* is used to describe a dying patient. It describes what is known as the "death rattle." Before suctioning was prevalent, fluids would gather in the lungs and make it difficult to breath. Because of this difficulty, patients at the end of life would emit a rattling sound from their chest during breathing.[362]
- Rabbi Moshe Feinstein writes that the prohibition to touch a *goseis* begins when the patient is at the point of *nutah la'mus* — beginning the actual dying process (i.e., organs shutting down, etc.).[363]
- As we mentioned previously, Rabbi Wosner writes that there is

361 *Yoma* 85a.

362 Rema, Even HaEzer 121:7.

363 *Igros Moshe*, Choshen Mishpat 2:73:3.

a doubt when exactly a patient gets the status of a *goseis*.[364]

- Is it permitted to touch or move the patient very gently? According to the Shach, a *goseis* may be moved slightly in order to remove an "impediment to the soul leaving."[365]
- In a similar vein, Rabbi Shlomo Zalman Auerbach has been quoted to permit patting an agitated patient who is a *goseis* to calm him or her.[366]
- Furthermore, the Talmud clearly indicates that minimizing pain and human dignity are both important concerns for a patient at the end of life.[367]

Conclusion

Based on these sources, it seems that if a dying patient's condition is presently stable,[368] it is not clear whether he has the status of a *goseis*. Therefore for the purpose of *kavod habrios*, the patient may be carefully and gently moved for cleaning. However, if the patient's condition is rapidly deteriorating, he probably has the status of a *goseis* and it is best not to touch him.

Resuscitation and Intubation in Halachah

Q: Is it permissible for a patient to refuse to be resuscitated or intubated (put on a respirator)?

A: There are different approaches to these issues. The Torah gives great value to every second of life and obligates us to seek

364 *Shevet HaLevi* 9:245.

365 *Nekudos HaKesef*, Yoreh Dei'ah 339:1; see also *Bais Lechem Yehudah*.

366 *Shulchan Shlomo*, Refuah 2, p. 23.

367 See *Sanhedrin* 45a.

368 Life support may also give the patient increased stability and make them less susceptible to be affected by being moved gently; see *Shulchan Shlomo* ibid.

medical attention. Nonetheless, there is discussion in classic and contemporary sources as to the extent of this obligation. We will consider two basic approaches to resuscitation and intubation.

The Talmud relates that when the great sage Rebbe Yehudah the Prince was suffering from his final illness, the rabbis gathered and prayed for him fervently. The servant of Rebbe saw his pain and purposely disrupted the rabbis' prayers in order to cause Rebbe's passing, which is what happened.[369] The Ran understands that the servant's behavior was proper. He uses this story as a source that if a person is terminally ill and in great pain, it is permissible to pray to Hashem to take them and end his suffering.[370] The Aruch HaShulchan cites the comments of the Ran as the halachah.

Rabbi Moshe Feinstein and other halachic authorities understand that the Ran's position is not limited to prayer and applies also to a patient refusing treatment.[371] According to the Ran, Rebbe was terminally ill and therefore his suffering was a consideration. They learn from here that in a case of terminal illness, certain treatments may be withheld in order to prevent prolonged suffering. Based on my discussions with Rabbi Feinstein's leading disciples,[372] it seems that there are two primary considerations: pain and consciousness. If a patient is clearly in pain, we are not obligated to give them medical attention that will prolong their suffering. Additionally, if the patient is in an irreversible coma, that may also be a reason not to prolong their illness.[373] According to this approach, the patient's wishes also play an important role in making these decisions.

With this in mind, we can now consider refusing resuscitation for a terminally ill patient. Some contemporary halachic authorities

---

369 *Kesubos* 104a.

370 *Nedarim* 40a.

371 *Igros Moshe* Choshen Mishpat 2:73–75; *Tiferes Yisrael*, *Yomah* 7 (Boaz 3); *Divrei Moshe* [Halberstam] 95; *Emek HaTeshuvah* 6:499.

372 See *Igros Moshe* ibid.; Rabbi Zev Schostack, *Journal of Halachah & Contemporary Society* XXII; *Tradition* 34:2, based on Rabbi Feinstein's approach; Rabbi Aharon Felder in *Reshumai Aharon*.

373 See Meiri quoted in Biur Halachah 329, and dispute between Beis Yaakov and Shevus Yaakov about desecrating Shabbos for a *goseis* cited in *Sha'arei Teshuvah*, Orach Chaim 329.

view the potential of breaking ribs,[374] and the poor prognosis of a patient who is resuscitated, as sufficient to refuse to be resuscitated.[375] However, intubation is considered less traumatic than resuscitation, although it is accompanied with discomfort and prolongs the illness. Therefore, if the patient specifically requested not to be intubated, we honor this request. Otherwise, we must assume that the patient's will is to be intubated unless there is great pain,[376] the patient is in an irreversible coma, or the patient's condition is too precarious to really be effective.[377]

Other contemporary authorities take a more limited view of the story of Rebbe.[378] They are not sure if all authorities agree with the Ran's acceptance of the actions of Rebbe's servant as the halachah. Furthermore, the Ran's comments may be limited to prayer but do not apply to refusing medical treatment.[379] They base this approach on a comment of the Issur VeHeter, a Rishon, cited in the *Biur Halachah*.[380] The Talmud writes that Shabbos is desecrated to remove a person from the rubble. The Issur VeHeter comments that this is even the case if the person is so injured that he can only live for a few minutes. Rabbi Elyashiv understood that this indicates that there is an obligation to prolong life even under these circumstances. According to this approach, it is only permitted to withhold treatment in very extenuating circumstances. As such, they do not consider resuscitation or intubation to be causing great pain. Therefore they maintain that a terminally ill patient

---

374 See also *Sanhedrin* 45a, which considers pain and disgrace to be legitimate considerations. Breaking bones can be considered an issue of disgrace as well as pain.

375 It would seem, according to Rashi's interpretation, that Rebbe Yehudah experienced great discomfort, not necessarily pain; the Ran however uses the wording "great pain."

376 Rabbi Dovid Feinstein, quoted by Rabbi Schostack in *Tradition loc. cit.*

377 See Rabbi Yechezkel Roth in *Emek HaTeshuvah*)6:499), who also permits withholding intubation in difficult situations based on the Ran.

378 See *Shiurim LeRofim* 3:189,190,192, by Rabbi Yitzchok Zilberstein, son-in-law of the late Rabbi Elyashiv.

379 See *Minchas Shlomo* 1:91:24. However, Rabbi Shmuel Wosner in *Shevet HaLevi* (2:179, 8:293) and *Divrei Moshe* (95) dismiss this correlation and argue that the Torah only gives permission to desecrate the Shabbos, but it is not necessarily obligatory.

380 Orach Chaim 329.

should be resuscitated or intubated in most situations.[381] Likewise they do not recognize a patient being in an irreversible coma as reason to withhold resuscitation or intubation.

Defining Life and Death

Q: How do halachic sources define death?

A: This is one of the most sensitive and complicated issues in the field of halachah and medicine. The intention of this discussion is not to offer any conclusive answers to these great questions. Rather, we will leave the conclusions to *gedolei olam*, the greatest Sages of our day, to decide. Here we will simply present some of the sources and discussion on this subject, which in the context of *lo l'halachah v'lo lema'aseh* — purely theoretical grounds, are fascinating.

The source material on this subject focuses on three aspects:

- Cessation of breathing
- Heartbeat
- Decapitation

Cessation of Breathing

A famous passage in *Yoma* states if a person is trapped under the rubble, we desecrate Shabbos in order to save him.[382] The rescuers should uncover the head until the nostrils and look for signs of breathing. The nostrils are viewed as the source of life, as the verse says "*kol asher nishmas chaim b'apo* — all who have life in their nostrils."[383] If the

---

381 *Nishmas Avraham*, Yoreh Dei'ah 339, quoting Rabbi Elyashiv.

382 83a, 85a.

383 *Bereishis* 20:22.

person is not breathing, the rescuers do not desecrate Shabbos further because it is assumed that he has died.

The Rambam writes in the laws of Shabbos: "A person who rubble fell on him... if they checked until his nostrils and they did not find breathing, they leave him there [until after Shabbos] because he has already died."[384] In the laws of mourning, the Rambam adds that before moving the body, "they should wait a little maybe he fainted [and is still alive]."[385]

The Chachmas Adom and *Kitzur Shulchan Aruch* write: "After the soul departs, a light feather is placed by the nostrils, if it does not move, it is known that the person has died."[386] Interestingly, *Nitei Gavriel*, a contemporary compendium on the laws of mourning, cites the custom of burial societies in Jerusalem to wait twenty or thirty minutes before placing the feather to verify death.

From these sources it seems that the main indicator of life or death is breathing. The primacy of breathing as the main indicator of life is underscored by the Chasam Sofer, who sought to dispel the notion that the halachic definition of death is not until the body begins to decompose. He writes that once breathing has stopped, a person is considered dead and it is prohibited for a Kohen to be in the same room. He sums up his position and writes: "however, after the body is resting like an inanimate stone and does not have any movement [lit. beating] and there is no breathing, we only have the words of our holy Torah that the person is considered dead."[387] It is important to note that on the one hand, the Chasam Sofer emphatically considers breathing to be the main criterion, yet he also seems to require cessation of all body movements, such as heartbeat, as well to determine death.

Heartbeat

The Chacham Tzvi was asked about a young woman who opened a slaughtered chicken and did not find a heart. Is the chicken considered

---

384 2:19.

385 4:5.

386 194:5.

387 *Shu"t*, Yoreh Dei'ah 338.

a *treifah* — an animal with a terminal ailment, and therefore not kosher?

He cites the comments of the Kesef Mishnah, who asks why the Rambam does not count a missing heart in his list of *treifos*. He answers that the Rambam omitted it because it is simply impossible for an animal to live without a heart. Therefore, it was not necessary for the Rambam to mention it. The Chacham Tzvi writes based on this idea, that it is impossible that the chicken did not have a heart, and as such we are compelled to assume that it must have had a heart before the slaughter but somehow got lost when the chicken was opened. Therefore the chicken is permitted. He emphatically supports the notion that it is impossible to live without a heart from the words of the *Zohar*, the Rambam in *Moreh Nevuchim*, and Rav Sa'adiah Gaon that the heart is the main organ of life and the dwelling place of the soul. He also understands that while breathing is important, this is because of its relationship to the functioning of the heart.[388] This responsa of the Chacham Tzvi and his sources are viewed as a strong indication that a beating heart is a sign of life.[389]

Similarly, in the late 1800s, the Maharsham was asked by a *chevrah kaddisha* for direction. They had buried a person after he had seemingly died. The members had checked the nostrils many times with a feather and did not find any breathing. However, some movement was felt in other areas of the body. The Maharsham felt that they acted incorrectly and needed atonement. He explained: "it is correct that the main source of living is in the nostrils (as the halachah states that we only check the nostrils of a person who is under rubble), however this is only a general rule.... However if they observe an indication of life in the other organs, we do not rely on the checking of the nostrils."[390]

Similarly, Rabbi Moshe Feinstein, in an early response in *Igros Moshe*, discusses if a patient is considered dead when there is no discernible breathing but the EKG indicates that the heart is beating. He contends

---

388 74:77.

389 See *Igros Moshe*, Yoreh Dei'ah 2:174, and *Minchas Yitzchak* (5:7–8) for further discussion of this point.

390 6:124.

that the person is still considered alive, even though it is not discernible to human senses without the aid of the machine.[391]

From these sources it seems that although breathing is the only sign mentioned in the Talmud, it is not the sole criterion. Therefore, if other body movements are detected, particularly a beating heart, the person is still considered living.

Artificial Breathing

With the advent of artificial respiration, a patient with no brain function and unable to breathe otherwise can still absorb enough oxygen to keep vital organs alive. This could allow the heart to still beat and even give birth. This condition is known as brain stem death. The stem of the brain that controls involuntary movements is dead, but because of artificial respiration the heart and other organs continue to function. This new phenomenon raises a perplexing question. If the only reason the heart is beating is because of artificial respiration, is this still considered a sign of life? Should these movements be viewed with the same significance as those mentioned by the Chasam Sofer, Maharsham, and *Igros Moshe*? In other words, is a person whose organs are functioning solely because of artificial respiration still considered alive?

The famous sheep experiment possibly indicates that the organ function caused by artificial respiration is not a significant sign of life. A pregnant sheep was put on a heart and lung machine and then decapitated. According to the Mishnah in *Oholos*, decapitation is a sure form of death.[392] Nonetheless, a live lamb was delivered through cesarean section. Live birth, according to the Talmud, is a proof of life.[393] How could there be a live birth if the sheep is halachically dead? This would seem to prove that live birth is only an indication of life when the mother is not connected to machines that artificially keep her alive. However, when she is being kept alive by artificial respiration, live birth is no longer a proof of life. In the same way, it could be argued that a heartbeat that

391 Yoreh Dei'ah 2:146.

392 1:6.

393 *Erchin* 7a.

is only the result of a respirator does not carry the same significance as the movements mentioned by the Chasam Sofer, Maharsham, and *Igros Moshe*. However, for many reasons, the sheep experiment is not a conclusive proof that brain stem death is recognized by halachah. It is only a proof that a decapitated animal whose heart is still beating is definitely considered dead. We will address the differences between the two later in our discussion.

Rabbi Sternbuch's Approach

Rabbi Moshe Sternbuch in *Teshuvos VeHanhagos* understands the intent of the Chasam Sofer to be that the fundamental sign of life is the ability to breathe. We see this clearly from the Talmud in *Yoma* quoted above that derives this from the verse in *Bereishis*. Rabbi Sternbuch understands that the concern about other movements mentioned by the Chasam Sofer is secondary. It is only because in a traditional setting it may indicate that the patient is still able to breathe. As such, in a situation of brain stem death where the ability for spontaneous respiration has been completely lost, the patient can be considered dead. The other movements are not true indicators of life. Therefore, once the loss of spontaneous respiration is verified we do not need to be concerned with these movements.[394]

This approach is a plausible explanation of Rabbi Feinstein's position on whether cessation of spontaneous respiration determines death even if the heart is beating. As mentioned previously, in an early responsum, Rabbi Feinstein was concerned about a heartbeat detected by an EKG even though the patient was not breathing, which seems to indicate that Rabbi Feinstein viewed heartbeat as a sign of life. However, in a responsum dated Iyar 1976, he considers spontaneous respiration for a person on a respirator to be the sole factor in determining death.[395] In a letter published in a later volume of *Igros Moshe*, Rabbi Feinstein writes: "although the heart could beat for a

---

394 4:268.

395 *Igros Moshe*, Yoreh Dei'ah 3:132, according to the understanding of his son Rabbi Dovid Feinstein, and grandson Rabbi Rappaport cited in *Assia*.

few days, nonetheless as long as the patient does not have the ability to breathe on its own, he is considered dead."[396]

The two statements of Rabbi Feinstein seem to contradict each other. Is breathing the only factor or is heartbeat also significant?

According to Rabbi Sternbuch's approach, it is possible that the earlier responsum was referring to a patient in a traditional setting. Cessation of breathing had been observed but the EKG signal indicated that normal organ functions had not completely ceased. Therefore it is possible that the patient may still have the ability to breathe, and as such we must be stringent. However, the later responsa were referring to a patient with brain stem death on a respirator. In this setting it is clear that there is no ability for spontaneous respiration and the organ function can be attributed to the artificial respiration. As such, the heartbeat does not have intrinsic significance. Therefore, we only follow the primary sign of life, which is spontaneous respiration.[397]

Multiple Signs

Rabbi Wosner in *Shevet HaLevi* understands that breathing is not the sole sign of life. He cites the *Zohar*, Rav Sa'adiah Gaon, Chacham Tzvi, Chasam Sofer, and Maharsham, who underscore the importance of the heart and other signs as well. Rabbi Wosner explains that although the Talmud in *Yoma* only mentions breathing, if there is a heartbeat, a person is considered living in all circumstances.[398] Rabbi Waldenberg in *Tzitz Eliezer* also quotes these sources and understands that life is not contingent on brain stem function. Therefore, if the heart is still functioning the person is considered living even if there is no spontaneous respiration.[399]

Rabbi Y. Zilberstein explains the position of Rabbi Yosef Shalom

---

396 Yoreh Dei'ah 4:54; see original in *Assia* XII.

397 In Cheshvan 1987, the Chief Rabbinate of Israel and Rabbi Shaul Yisraeli recognized brain stem death as a halachic definition of death. Their position was largely based on the understanding that breathing is the sole factor in determining death. See *Assia* XII for a full discussion on the position of the Chief Rabbinate.

398 7:235.

399 18:66.

Elyashiv about this point. Rabbi Elyashiv viewed heartbeat as an independent sign of life. However, he pointed out that in theory a heart that is beating artificially is not a sign of life. This can be demonstrated by the fact that even a heart that has been removed from the body can still beat (!). Clearly, the heart is not alive. Nonetheless, Rabbi Elyashiv still viewed the heartbeat of a patient with brain stem death as a possible sign of life. He was concerned that the heart could still beat on its own. Therefore, even if there is no spontaneous respiration, this concern would deter us from considering the patient to be dead.[400]

Challenges in Verifying Cessation of Breathing

We have learned that there is a difference of opinion if breathing is the sole sign of life. Nonetheless, even if it is the sole criterion, there are challenges in implementing this approach. How do we verify that the person has stopped breathing? Clinically, this can be done by temporarily disconnecting the respirator and observing if there is any breathing for eight to ten minutes. This is called the apnea test. However, there are two halachic issues with this test.

In the 1976 responsum in *Igros Moshe*, Rabbi Feinstein describes a respirator connected to an oxygen tank. He writes: "as long as the machine is working, it is prohibited to remove it because maybe he is living and will die because of this. However, when the oxygen supply is finished, they should not reconnect the machine again until they wait a short period of time, like fifteen minutes. If he is not alive there will be no breathing and they will know that he is dead."[401] We can learn from here that there are two possible issues with the apnea test:

- The patient cannot be removed from a respirator for the apnea test because if the person is still alive this may cause him to die, or at least hasten death.
- The amount of time used for the apnea test is less than the accepted practice of the *chevrah kaddisha*. It is customary for the *chevrah kaddisha* to observe no movement for fifteen to thirty minutes. However, when conducting the apnea test,

400 *Shiurei Torah LeRofim* 2:145.

401 Yoreh Dei'ah 3:132.

the patient is only observed for less than ten minutes. Rabbi Shlomo Zalman Auerbach points out that before ample time has elapsed, there is still a *sofek* — halachic doubt, if the person is living.

Decapitation

The Rambam writes: "A dead body does not contract ritual impurity until the soul departs, even severely wounded or near death [*goseis*]... [however] if the neck was broken with most of the flesh, or ripped like a fish from the back, or decapitated or divided into two from the abdomen, this gives off ritual impurity although there is movement in one of the limbs."[402] According to halachah, decapitation is a clear sign of death. Could brain stem death be compared to decapitation? Is actual decapitation required to be considered death, or is the cessation of brain function sufficient?

Rabbi Shlomo Zalman Auerbach wrote: "fundamentally, a person whose entire brain is irreversibly dead to the point that there is not a single living cell in the brain, it is possible that he is dead, even if his heart is beating because of a ventilator... because in this situation the body is just an incubator."[403] At least in theory, Rabbi Auerbach agreed that a brain without any function and decapitation are synonymous.

However, Rabbi Yosef Shalom Elyashiv, cited by Rabbi Y. Zilberstein disagreed. He understood that the Rambam is only referring to actual decapitation. Complete death of the brain is not the same thing as decapitation.[404]

Rabbi Feinstein in *Igros Moshe* touches upon this point in his discussion about the blood flow test, a way of determining if there is blood flow to the brain. A radioactive dye is injected into the blood and observed on a scan. If there is no blood flow to the brain, it is presumed that the brain stem cells are dead because they have no supply of oxygen. He writes, "if this [the dye] does not come to the brain, it is clear that

402 *Mishneh Torah*, Tumas Meis 1:15, based on *Oholos* 1:6.

403 *Shulchan Shlomo*, Refuah; *Minchas Shlomo* 2.

404 *Shiurei Torah LeRofim* 2:145, footnotes 3–4.

the brain has no more connection to the body and it is also completely rotten and is like the head was decapitated."[405]

We can learn two points from Rabbi Feinstein's comments. Firstly, Rabbi Feinstein does not require actual decapitation. Secondly, he describes the brain as being completely rotten. This seems to indicate that he requires serious structural damage, not simply a pathological determination of cell death.[406] As such, the blood flow test may not be sufficient because it does not necessarily demonstrate complete degeneration of brain tissue.[407]

Another issue raised about using the blood flow test is if it is permitted to inject the dye into a patient that may be a *goseis*. Rabbi Moshe Sherer of Agudath Israel of America recorded in his diary a conversation that he had with Rabbi Feinstein on May 12, 1976, in which he asked whether a blood flow test has any significance for a patient breathing through a respirator. "Rabbi Feinstein replied, 'definitely not... the test cannot be performed altogether since the person is after all a *goseis*.' "[408] Rabbi Shlomo Zalman Auerbach also raised this issue.

Rabbi J. D. Bleich points out that many functions regulated by the brain stem are still present in patients with clinical brain death.[409] Along the same lines, Rabbi Shlomo Zalman Auerbach felt strongly that the blood flow test does not convincingly demonstrate that there is complete cell death, which was his criterion. As such, he still considered a patient who underwent the blood flow test to have the status of *sofek chai* — possibly living. He issued a joint statement with Rabbi

---

405 Yoreh Dei'ah 3:132.

406 It is interesting to note that in halachah we find a difference between paralysis and *yavesh ka'eitz* — dryed out like a piece of wood.

407 While the teshuvah in *Igros Moshe* recommends using the blood flow test to verify brain death, it was in a situation where cessation of breathing was already verified by visual observation for fifteen minutes. Rabbi Feinstein writes that "since you say that now there is a test that great doctors could verify by injecting a solution into the body [i.e., blood flow test]... we should be stringent and not decide the patient to be dead before they do this test." The question becomes if the blood flow test could be relied on alone without the traditional observation of cessation of breathing. Furthermore, it is questionable if it is permitted to inject the solution into a patient that may still be alive but is a *goseis*.

408 *Rabbi Sherer* (Mesorah Publications), p. 492, note 12.

409 See Rabbi Bleich's *Time of Death in Halachah*.

Elyashiv against recognizing brain death. On the other hand, the former Sephardic Chief Rabbi, Rabbi Shlomo Amar, and Rabbi Ovadia Yosef ruled that on a case-by-case basis, with proper rabbinic oversight, brain stem death could be accepted in order to permit heart transplants.[410]

The Heart and Lung Machine in Halachah

Q: Does halachah view a person on a heart and lung machine as living, considering that there is no breathing or heartbeat?

A: This is an intriguing question with many ramifications in halachah. We will begin with an important seventeenth century discussion in the laws of *treifos*. We will then develop its relevance to contemporary questions about heart and lung machines.

Dispute over a Heartless Chicken

The *Shulchan Aruch* writes that an animal missing its heart is a *treifah* and not kosher.[411] The Kesef Mishnah explains why the Rambam does not mention a missing heart when he lists the ailments that render an animal a *treifah*. He writes: "the Rambam only mentions maladies of organs that, if missing or damaged, the animal could still live for a short amount of time. However, the Rambam did not list organs that if missing or removed the animal could not survive even for a short amount of time. These would be considered a *neveilah* — already dead. Likewise, an organ that an animal could not be born without, like a brain, heart,

410 For an extensive discussion of Rabbi Ovadia Yosef's position on brain stem death, see *Ruach Yaakov*, written by a grandson.

411 Yoreh Dei'ah 40:5.

esophagus, or trachea, he did not mention because they do not occur."[412]

As we mentioned briefly in our previous discussion, the Chacham Tzvi was asked about a slaughtered chicken where no heart was found inside. Curiously, the Chacham Tzvi ruled that the chicken is kosher despite the *Shulchan Aruch's* ruling that an animal missing a heart is a *treifah*.[413] He made an interesting argument. Since the Kesef Mishnah wrote that it is impossible for the chicken to have been living without a heart, there had to have been a heart. It must have fallen out when the chicken was opened and was eaten by an eager house cat. As such, the chicken is kosher. The Chacham Tzvi wrote that even if witnesses testify that there was no heart, we should consider them to be lying rather than accept the impossibility of a "heartless" living chicken! The Chacham Tzvi cited additional proofs from the *Zohar*, *Moreh Nevuchim*, and Rav Sa'adiah Gaon, all saying that the source of life is in the heart and therefore it is preposterous to maintain that the chicken could be living without a heart.

The *Kraisi U'Plaisi*, written by Rabbi Yehonasan Eybeshitz, felt the Chacham Tzvi had gone too far. Rabbi Eybeshitz agreed that in the original case of the heartless chicken, it is most probable that there was a heart and it was snatched by the hungry house cat. However, he was skeptical of rendering the chicken kosher against the words of two competent witnesses. Rabbi Eybeshitz questioned how the Chacham Tzvi was so sure that it is completely impossible. He pointed out that the Rambam only omitted this case but did not go so far as to say it is like a dead carcass. This could be because the Rambam did not want to completely rely on his own logical conclusion that it is an impossibility. Therefore, the safer approach would be to consider the chicken not kosher.[414]

Heart Transplantation

Halachic discussion about the permissibility of heart transplants began when it was a new concept with very poor success rates. One issue

---

412 See *Mishneh Torah*, Shechitah 10:9.

413 74, 77.

414 Interestingly, the *Kraisi U'Plaisi* cited a report from physicians of his time that perhaps other organs could compensate for the heart. It is also possible that the chicken had a heart but was malformed.

raised was how the heart could be harvested from a donor who may be halachically considered living. That was the subject of our discussion about brain stem death. However, there was an interesting argument raised to prohibit receiving a heart transplant as well. In order to receive the transplant, the recipient's original heart must be removed. If a person without a heart is considered dead, the patient is being "killed" in order to receive the new heart. This raises a fundamental problem. If a stopped or missing heart is halachically viewed as death, how could recipients allow their heart to be removed? Is it permitted to "die" in order to live?

The divergent views of the Chacham Tzvi and *Kraisi U'Plaisi* became a focal point in this discussion. According to the Chacham Tzvi, a heart that is missing is a sure sign of halachic death. Therefore immediately when the recipient's heart is removed in preparation for the transplant he should be considered dead. The patient's subsequent "revival" after the new heart is implanted could be viewed as a "resurrection"! If this is correct, it would be highly questionable if a patient is permitted to "die" in order to live a longer life.[415] However, according to the *Kraisi U'Plaisi*, missing a heart is not an inherent sign of death. Therefore, if the patient's life is being maintained throughout the transplant by a heart and lung machine, we can consider him to be very much alive.

Heartless Widow?

Rabbi Menachem Kasher in *Divrei Menachem* pointed out that the implications of applying the logic of the Chacham Tzvi to heart transplants are very far-reaching. If a husband undergoing the surgery is considered halachically dead during the surgery, his wife would then be a widow. If so, after he becomes "resurrected" with his new heart, he would have to remarry his own wife![416] Furthermore, Rabbi Yisrael Meir

415 The objection of the *Igros Moshe* to be a recipient of a heart transplant (Yoreh Dei'ah 2:174, Choshen Mishpat 2:72) in the letters from 1968 and 1978, respectively, considering heart transplants as "murder of two souls" was because of the very poor outcomes, not because it is fundamentally forbidden to remove one's heart to receive a transplant. However, the *Minchas Yitzchak* 5:7, and *Tzitz Eliezer* 10:25:5–6, 17:66:1–2 raised this issue more earnestly.

416 *Shu"t* 1:27.

Lau in *Yachel Yisrael* points out that there is no real difference between a heart transplant or open heart surgery. During open heart surgery, the regular beating of the heart is interrupted and the patient is arguably "dead," and yet no one has prohibited such procedures on these grounds.[417]

While there may be various solutions to this halachic problem,[418] I would like to propose a solution of my own.

Rabbi Emden's Approach

The son of the Chacham Tzvi, Rabbi Yaakov Emden, sought to alleviate some of the criticism of his father's position on the heartless chicken. He explains in *Sheilas Yaavetz* that even though his father asserted that the witnesses are not believed, it is not because it is a total impossibility. Rather, it would be considered *ma'aseh nissim* — a miraculous occurrence. While we believe miracles can happen, the remoteness of the possibility makes it more probable that the witnesses are lying.[419]

According to Rabbi Emden's understanding of his father's position, he is conceding that a heartless chicken is not fundamentally dead. Rather it would be a rare and miraculous occurrence for a chicken to be living without a heart. This could mean that a missing heart is different from other forms of death, like decapitation. A decapitated person is considered dead even if the headless body could miraculously walk and function (!). On the other hand, a person missing a heart is assumed to have died, but if he is functioning, he is still alive.

Based on this new understanding of the Chacham Tzvi, we could reconsider the status of a person attached to a heart and lung machine. Living without a heart is not the same as decapitation. They don't *have* to be dead, but they are just probably dead. As such, if medicine has developed a machine that supports life without a heart, halachah could recognize them as being living. It just may be considered miraculous,

---

417 *Yachel Yisrael* 2:84.

418 See *Divrei Menachem* and *Yachel Yisrael* ibid. for further discussion.

419 1:121.

ma'aseh nissim. It would also seem that according to Rabbi Emden, his father's reference to the *Zohar* and other sources is to indicate that the heart as the center of life is a general idea but subject to exception.

Defining Miraculous

As we have learned, Rabbi Emden considers living without a heart as miraculous. However, it would seem that this does not apply to a person living on a heart and lung machine. Once the technology exists, it is a new reality and is quite "normal."

There is a related discussion among contemporary *poskim* about the concept of *ma'aseh nissim*, viewing an event as improbable and miraculous. There is a question whether an infant conceived via artificial insemination can be circumcised on Shabbos. The basic discussion revolves around the comments of Rabbeinu Chananel, who wrote that if a woman conceives "artificially" by being inseminated through sitting in a bath, it is considered *ma'aseh nissim* and Shabbos cannot be desecrated to perform the circumcision. This is because a circumcision is not performed on Shabbos when the conception or the birth is not natural. Rabbi Shlomo Zalman Auerbach argued that today's artificial reproductive technologies may have the same status. However, Rabbi Shmuel Wosner in *Shevet HaLevi* strongly dismissed this notion, writing that we cannot consider these commonplace procedures as *ma'aseh nissim*, and therefore artificial conception is considered normal and the bris can be performed on Shabbos.[420] Rabbi Wosner explained that we cannot compare artificial reproductive technologies to the improbable methods mentioned by Rabbeinu Chananel. Rabbeinu Chananel's case was a rare and miraculous occurrence, very different from the highly developed reproductive technologies of today. They are not miraculous but a new reality.

In a similar vein, Rabbi Moshe Feinstein writes that in the laws of *treifos*, an animal that survived a commonplace surgery cannot be called *ma'aseh nissim* (see footnote for discussion).[421] This fits very well

420 9:209.

421 Rabbi Feinstein maintains that the definition of *treifos* in the laws of kashrus is fixed on the mortality of these maladies at the time of the giving of the Torah on Sinai. However, the definition of *treifos* for criminal punishment depends on the mortality rate in contemporary

with Rabbi Wosner's approach. They both agree that a commonplace medical intervention becomes a new reality and is no longer considered miraculous.

Conclusion

Based on these sources, we could arrive at the following conclusions:

- The Kesef Mishnah and Chacham Tzvi, who viewed a heartless chicken as dead, were referring to a chicken living without a heart at all. However, as qualified by Rabbi Emden, the Chacham Tzvi never considered missing a heart as a fundamental sign of death like decapitation. Rather, it is highly improbable and miraculous.
- The new phenomena of living on a heart and lung machine during an open heart surgery or transplant is quite different from Rabbi Emden's discussion of the heartless chicken. The very fact that these procedures are commonplace with high success rates forces us to recognize these situations as a new reality. This is similar to how Rabbi Wosner recognized artificial insemination to be different than Rabbeinu Chananel's comments about an artificial pregnancy.
- Therefore, although many sources consider the heart as the home of the soul, this is only as a general rule when the heart is removed. A person on a heart and lung machine is entirely different. Under these unique conditions, we can consider the patient to be living, albeit without a heart.
- Additionally, it could be argued that the machine can be viewed as part of the patient's body and therefore the patient is not completely "without" a heart.
- Therefore, we will not view stopping the heart for a transplant

---

times (*Igros Moshe*, Even HaEzer 2:3:2, Yoreh Dei'ah 3:33, Choshen Mishpat 73:4). To arrive at this conclusion he asserts that the Sages recognized that nature changes and that these occurrences of survival cannot be dismissed as *ma'aseh nissim*. Therefore, the definition of a *treifah* for kashrus must be fixed, based on the conditions at the time of the giving of the Torah. In his discussion he writes: "today this surgery has been done to millions [of people and animals, and they lived] and certainly it can not be considered a miracle or a minority" (Even HaEzer loc. cit.). The Chazon Ish arrived at the same conclusion.

or heart surgery as an act of murder. As such, we can consider a patient on a heart and lung machine to be very much alive — and married!

Washing Hands after Touching the Dead

Q: A physician's assistant sometimes has to pronounce the death of a patient, which includes physical contact with the deceased. What is the halachah regarding washing hands afterward? Should the PA get a washing cup and wash as one does in the morning? Should the cup be turned upside down afterward like the custom is to do after a funeral? Is there a difference if the patient is Jewish or not?

A: Here is an overview of the issues involved:

The *Shulchan Aruch* writes that hands should be washed after touching a dead person.[422] According to the Magen Avraham, this washing does not need to be with a cup or three times as is done in the morning. However, other sources require a cup and three times and there are varying customs.[423] Additionally, it is unclear if there is any obligation to wash if the deceased person was not Jewish.[424] Likewise, there may not be an obligation to wash if the caretaker's hands were gloved.

The common custom after a funeral is to wash hands three times with a cup and turn the cup over. However, it is unclear if these customs apply to all situations where people are in the presence of a deceased

422 Orach Chaim 4:18.

423 See *Piskei Teshuvos* for extensive sources.

424 *Yad HaLevi* cited in *Piskei Teshuvos*.

person. In addition, the custom of turning over the cup may not have a strong source.[425]

- In summation, the main obligation is to wash the hands, even without a cup. Therefore, if a cup is available, it is a plus. However, even if there is no cup available one should still wash. If the patient was not Jewish or the attendant was wearing gloves, there is more of a reason to be lenient.
- If the hands can be washed with a cup, at least before coming in contact with food, that would be best.
- It does not seem necessary to turn over the cup in a hospital setting. This is because it is unclear if the custom is only after a funeral and we generally do not extend these customs when in doubt.

Organ Transplantation vs. the Mitzvah of Burial

Q: There is a prohibition to derive benefit from the body of a deceased person. There is also a great mitzvah to bury the dead. Does removing an organ for a transplant violate this prohibition? Is this considered neglecting the obligation to bury the dead?

A: This is a complex subject:

Is a Transplanted Organ Considered Alive?

The book of Kings tells the story of the son of the Shunamis who

425 See *Piskei Teshuvos* who cites sources that question the origin of the custom not to dry the hands. The same may be true with this custom as well.

died and was resurrected by the prophet Elisha. The Talmud asks a most interesting question. Since the child died and was therefore *tamei meis* — had the ritual impurity of a dead body — did he still have the status of a corpse and emit ritual impurity once Elisha brought him back to life? The Talmud answers, "Rabbi Yeshoshua said the dead give off impurity, not the living." Meaning to say, if the boy is living he cannot have the status of a corpse that emits *tumah*.[426]

Based on this passage, Rabbi Unterman argued that a transplanted organ regains its living status and no longer emits ritual impurity. As such, he extends this logic to the prohibition to derive benefit from the dead and the obligation to bury the deceased. Since the organ regains its living status, there is no obligation of burial or prohibition to derive benefit from it.[427]

Esrog Branches and Grafting

Another possible basis for this approach is a Talmudic passage in *Sotah*.[428] The Talmud is discussing the laws of *orlah*, the prohibition to benefit from the fruits of a tree during its first three years. The Talmud deals with an interesting question. If the branch from a young tree is grafted to an old tree (or vice versa), does it retain its own status or does it get the status of the host tree? The Talmud contends that the branch gets the status of the host tree for the laws of *orlah*. This means that if the host tree is older, the fruits growing from a young grafted branch are permitted. Rashi explains that the branch becomes *batel* — insignificant, in relation to the tree.

This passage became an important source about whether *esrogim*

---

426 *Niddah* 70b.

427 Rabbi Malkiel Tenenbaum, in *Divrei Malkiel* 4:97, raises a similar point. The Talmud considers an infant that was born prematurely and has no chance of survival as "not living." As such, can a Kohen, who is prohibited from being in the same room as a deceased person, be in the same room as the premature infant?
Rabbi Tennenbaum understands that although the infant does not have the status of living, since at that moment it is very much alive, it does not give off *tumah*. Therefore a Kohen can stay in the room. In a similar vein, one could raise the point along the lines of Rabbi Unterman that if the organ is functioning it must be considered "alive."

428 43b.

from a grafted tree may be used for Succos. If an *esrog* branch is grafted on to a lemon tree, is the fruit considered an *esrog* or a lemon? Based on this concept, the branch should get the status of the host. Therefore it has the status of a lemon and is not acceptable for Succos.

A transplanted limb may be similar to the branch grafted onto a tree. Just as the branch gets the status of the tree, so too the organ should be considered part of the recipient's body. This would let us consider the organ to still be "living." As such, there may be no obligation to bury the organ nor a restriction to derive benefit from it.[429]

Rav Ovadia's View

Rabbi Ovadia Yosef in *Yabia Omer* discusses this argument in his correspondence with his lifelong friend Rabbi Ben Tzion Abba Shaul about cornea donation.[430] Rabbi Yosef points out that the Talmud's comments about the story of the son of the Shunamis were dealing with ritual impurity. However, it may not be a conclusive proof for questions about deriving benefit from the deceased and the obligation of burial. For this reason, Rabbi Yosef was not comfortable relying on Rabbi Unterman's logic alone. Therefore, Rabbi Yosef raised additional reasons to be lenient:

- Mitzvah to bury the dead: It is not clear whether the obligation to bury a limb is a Torah obligation or rabbinic. Because it is possible that this is not a question of a Torah prohibition it would be easier to rely on Rabbi Unterman's logic.
- Deriving benefit from the dead: Generally forms of benefit that are prohibited by the Torah are only prohibited when the benefit is enjoyed in a normal manner. This is called *derech hana'ah*. If the benefit is not received in a normal way, it may be more lenient. This concept is called *shelo kiderech hana'ah* — deriving benefit in an unusual way. Rabbi Yosef asserts that according

429 This is similar to Rabbi Moshe Feinstein's reasoning in the next discussion as to why a transplanted organ does not give off *tumah*. Rabbi Feinstein considered it to be *batel* — nullified, because it is being used for a new purpose.

430 *Yabia Omer* 3, Yoreh Dei'ah 20–22.

to a number of opinions, deriving benefit from the dead body in an unusual manner is not a Torah prohibition. Furthermore, he argues that the benefit derived from a transplanted organ is not considered a normal form of benefit and as such is not a Torah prohibition.

Kohen Receiving an Organ Transplant

Q: Is it permitted for a Kohen to receive an organ transplant from a deceased person?

A: A Kohen is not allowed to come in direct contact with a deceased person, which includes organs as well. By accepting the transplant, a patient who is a Kohen will be in direct contact with the organ all the time. With the advent of organ transplantation, contemporary halachic authorities looked to clarify this question and not simply rely on reasons of *pikuach nefesh*. Here is an overview of this most interesting discussion.

Tumah inside the Body

In the late 1950s, when the entire concept of organ transplantation was in its infancy, Rabbi Yitzchak Isaac Leibes, a distinguished European rabbi living in New York, wrote a treatise on potential halachic questions about the novel concept of transplantation. In his work *Kuntres Rofe Kol Bassar*, he dealt with many possible issues, including deriving benefit from a deceased person's body, Kohen issues, as well as the possible ramifications of transplanting reproductive organs. (Interestingly, some of the concepts could be applied to egg donation and surrogacy). In a twenty-page response dated Rosh Chodesh Av 5718 (1958), Rabbi

Moshe Feinstein, a contemporary of Rabbi Leibes, reviewed many of the arguments made in *Kuntres Rofe Kol Bassar* and offered his own perspective as well.[431]

One of the issues that Rabbi Leibes and Rabbi Feinstein discussed was our question about the permissibility of a Kohen to receive an organ transplant. Rabbi Leibes pointed out that if the size of the tissue being transplanted is more than an olive, it could give off *tumah* — ritual impurity, and a Kohen would be prohibited from coming in contact with it even in today's times. Rabbi Leibes offered a number of possible arguments to permit a Kohen to accept a transplant, such as relying on less mainstream opinions that maintain that there is not a Torah prohibition for a Kohen to defile himself in contemporary times when he is already ritually impure, as well as the opinion of the Maharashdam that questions the reliability of a Kohen's tradition on his lineage. Rabbi Feinstein did not view these reasons as being substantial, and offered a perspective of his own.

Firstly, Rabbi Feinstein pointed out that if the tissue will be put inside the body, there is a concept of *tumah balu'ah* — that ritual impurity is not transferred from inside the body. The commentary of Rabbeinu Shimshon explains that since it is inside the body, it loses its own significance and is considered a part of the body. Based on this idea, if the tissue is transplanted beneath the skin, the patient will not become *tamei* since it is not in contact with the external part of the recipient's body. This would be a significant argument to permit a Kohen to receive a transplant since most transplanted organs are not visible externally.

Furthermore, the Rambam writes that although human skin from a deceased person is ritually impure, if it is chemically treated it loses its *tumah*. The reason seems to be because when an item takes on a new form, it loses its previous status. Based on this concept, Rabbi Feinstein understands that if tissue from the deceased takes on a new role, like being used in a transplant, it removes the *tumah* status from it. As such, a Kohen would be allowed to accept a transplant (given certain

431 *Igros Moshe*, Yoreh Dei'ah 1:230.

provisions) even if it is not beneath the skin, because the very fact that it is now part of a living person gives it a new status and removes the *tumah*.

Kohen under Anesthesia

Rabbi Leibes raises a technical problem. How can the Kohen receive the transplant when he will contract *tumah* by being with the organ in the operating room until it is implanted into his body? Rabbi Leibes makes an interesting argument. Since the patient is under anesthesia during the operation, he should not have a prohibition to become *tamei* in that unconscious state. He is similar to a person who is mentally incapacitated and is not responsible for his mitzvah observance.

Rabbi Feinstein disagreed with this approach. He explains that a sleeping person is only exempt from mitzvos if he is an *ones* — beyond his control. However, in a situation where a person willingly goes into surgery, he has chosen a course of action and is responsible for what happens when he is sleeping. The only exemption would be if the person's state of unconsciousness is irreversible without outside intervention, which would make it a more permanent status than a person who is sleeping. In that situation, the person's status would change and could be considered a *shoteh* — a person without proper mental capacity, even if it was willfully induced.

Based on this differentiation, Rabbi Feinstein explains that a state of unconsciousness induced by anesthesia would only render a person a *shoteh* if medical intervention is needed in order to arouse the patient. However, since the anesthesia wears off on its own if not continuously induced, the patient would not have the status of a *shoteh*, but rather that of a sleeping person. As such, he is responsible if he comes in contact with *tumah* while unconscious.

Final Point

As a final thought, generally organ transplants are done to deal with life-threatening illnesses and therefore on a practical level, a Kohen would be allowed to accept the transplant regardless. Nonetheless, according to Rabbi Feinstein, if done with certain provisions, transplantation would not pose a halachic problem for a Kohen since the organ becomes a part of his body.

A Patient Who Was Unable to Sit Shivah

Q: An ill person was informed that a close relative passed away, but because of the patient's weakened state, he was unable to observe the laws of shivah properly, such as sitting on a low bench etc. When the person becomes stronger, does he need to observe shivah at that point similar to a person who did not know of his relative's passing, who must observe shivah when he is informed?

A: Interestingly, this important question was not directly discussed in *poskim* until a hundred years after the *Shulchan Aruch* was written. Here are some important points:

- Rabbi Shmuel HaLevi (1600s) was a student of the Taz. In his work *Nachlas Shivah*, he addresses the following question: if part or all of shivah was not observed fully, does the person need to start from the beginning when he becomes able to observe the laws of shivah? He writes that it is similar to a situation where shivah was not observed because one was unaware of the relative's passing. The halachah is that one is obligated to observe shivah when he finds out.[432] Likewise, in our situation, although he was aware of the relative's passing, the obligation of shivah was not fulfilled. As such, he must observe shivah

432 #17.

now. In a different responsum, the Nachlas Shivah cites a ruling from the great "Rabbi Shimon of Prague" taking this approach.[433] Many notable Acharonim, like the Chasam Sofer, Rabbi Shlomo Kluger, and Shoel U'Mashiv, concur with this opinion.[434]

- Rabbi Yaakov Reischer, the Rav of Prague, Worms, and Metz in the late 1600s and early 1700s, disagreed with the Nachlas Shivah in his classic responsa *Shevus Yaakov*. There Rabbi Reicher writes that there is an important difference between the case where the patient was unaware of the relative's passing and our case where the person was aware but was unable to observe shivah. He contends that the ruling of the great Rabbi Shimon of Prague was only given when the patient was completely unaware of what had happened. The difference is as follows — if the person was completely unaware of the loss, then obviously shivah was not observed in any form, however, if the patient was aware, it can be assumed that shivah was observed at least at some level, possibly by refraining from listening to music, beautification, or simply agonizing over the loss. According to this approach, these minor expressions of mourning are enough to be considered that shivah was observed and the patient would not have to observe shivah again. The Aruch HaShulchan, *Kitzur Shulchan Aruch*, *Mishnah Berurah*, and *Gesher HaChaim* agree with this approach. The *Teshuvah MeAhavah* writes that this was common practice.
- Rabbi Yitzchak Isaac Leibes (1906–2000), a distinguished contemporary rabbi and *posek*, was asked in 1959 about a woman whose mother passed away while she was in the hospital after childbirth. She could not observe the first few days of shivah fully but avoided listening to music and beautification. Rabbi Leibes cited the dispute between the *Nachlas Shivah* and *Shevus Yaakov* whether the days partially observed in the hospital would count. He concluded that she does not have to sit shivah

433 #73.

434 See *Nitei Gavriel* ch. 113 for all sources.

for any additional days based on the principle of *halachah kidivrei hameikil be'aveilus* — in the laws of mourning we generally follow the lenient opinion.[435] *Nitei Gavriel*, a contemporary work on the laws of mourning, also maintains that common practice is to follow the lenient opinion regarding a person who was aware that a relative passed away but was unable to fully observe the laws of shivah.

- All *poskim* agree that if the patient was aware of the loss then the obligation to tear *kri'ah* is only during the shivah period. The reason is because *kri'ah* is only performed *bisha'as chimum* — at the time when the emotions are still strong. This period is defined as the first seven days. If the person was not aware of the loss, then they are obligated to tear *kri'ah* for a relative if it is within thirty days of the passing. However, *kri'ah* is always performed for a parent.

---

435 *Beis Ovi* 1:97. He notes that although there is discussion as to how far reaching this principle is, in this situation where some of the laws of shivah were definitely observed, the lenient opinions could be relied upon.

EPILOGUE

It is appropriate to conclude with the directive of *Pirkei Avos*: "*Hafoch bah ve'hafoch bah dekulah bah* — continuously toil in Torah because all knowledge is in it." The profundity of the Torah is only exposed through tireless study and erudition. As the fields of medicine and mental health rapidly develop, we are constantly faced with new challenges and dilemmas. We intuitively know that the Torah can guide us and illuminate these challenges and opportunities. However, that light is not always so apparent and clear. Our Sages' directive of "*Hafoch bah ve'hafoch bah*" provides an answer. It is only through continuous study and devotion that we can find the halachic parallels we need to direct us how to view each new situation. If we are satisfied with superficial comparisons and haphazard answers, we sacrifice the profundity of what the Torah truly has to offer.

The Torah instructs us: "*Zechor yemos olam* — Remember the days of the world."[436] If we reach back into the great bygone eras of Torah scholarship, from Izmir to Lemberg, from Italy to Russia, from Eastern Europe to Northern Africa, from Eretz Yisrael to Bavel, we will find rich and fertile ground to build great intellectual edifices upon. If we care deeply about Torah and appreciate what the exciting fields of medicine and mental health have to offer, we can reach conclusions that will truly make the Torah great.

This work is a humble contribution to this lofty goal. I welcome you

---

436 *Devarim* 32:7.

to outdo me in both research and study. Feel free to disagree with my conclusions or comparisons. I will be honored that my work has helped others bring us closer to our deepest desire "*l'sakein olam be'malchus Shakai* — to perfect the world with Hashem's Kingship."

I invite you to join us as we continue this journey with the Medical Halachah Email for Professionals. If you are interested in receiving our posts, please send a request with your name and professional background to MedicalHalachaforProfessionals@Gmail.com.

IMPORTANT TERMS AND CONCEPTS

Acharonim Literally "the later ones," refers to Torah scholars from around 1500 CE to the present. Some notable Acharonim were Rabbi Yosef Karo and Rabbi Moshe Isserles (Rema), the authors of the *Shulchan Aruch*, Nodah BeYehudah, Rabbi Akiva Eiger, and Chasam Sofer.

agunah A woman whose husband disappeared and is unable to remarry.

chazakah A halachic assumption of status, often determined based on a previous status or a pattern of behavior.

chilul Shabbos Desecration of Shabbos.

choleh Ill person.

choleh sheyeish bo sakanah Illness with risk to life.

eino miskavein Literally "without intention," refers to an action that may inadvertently cause a transgression. Usually used in the laws of

	Shabbos.
goseis	Patient near death.
heter	A halachic leniency.
lifnei iver	Causing a person (Jew or non-Jew) to transgress the Torah.
melachos	The thirty-nine types of work forbidden to do on Shabbos. It is derived from the types of craftsmanship needed to build the Mishkan.
misayeia	Aiding a Jew in transgressing the Torah.
Mishkan	Tabernacle.
nefel	Literally refers to a stillborn fetus. Can also refer to an infant that cannot survive more than a short amount of time after birth, possibly thirty days.
pikuach nefesh	Saving a life. Refers to the concept that Torah prohibitions are suspended when there is a risk to life (except for the three cardinal sins).
psak	A halachic decision.
psik raisha	An unintentional action that will definitely cause a transgression. Usually used in the laws of Shabbos.
posek	Literally "a decider," a halachic decision maker.
Rishonim	Literally "the early ones," refers to Torah scholars from after the Geonim into the Middle Ages (approx. 1000–1500 CE). Some of the major Rishonim were Rashi, Rif, Tosfos, Rambam, Ramban, Rashba, Ritva, Rosh, Tur.
shailos v'teshuvos (Shu"t)	Rabbinic responsa.
sakanah	Risk to human life.
sofek	Doubt.

tomim tihiyeh — The commandment to walk simply before G-d and not overspeculate about the future.

tamei — Ritually impure.

treifah — An animal with a lethal condition specified in the laws of *treifos*. Usually cannot survive for twelve months. Can also refer to a lethal condition in humans.

yichud — The prohibition for an unmarried man and woman to be secluded together.

BIBLIOGRAPHY OF PRIMARY HALACHIC WORKS AND THEIR AUTHORS

Shulchan Aruch – Rabbi Yosef Karo was born in Toledo, Spain, in 1488, and passed away in Safed, Israel, in 1575. He left Spain in 1492 as a result of the Spanish expulsion of the Jews, and eventually became the Chief Rabbi of Safed. His magnum opus was the *Beis Yosef*, an encyclopedic commentary on the Tur. The halachic decisions were codified in the *Shulchan Aruch*. This work quickly became accepted throughout the Jewish world as authoritative. Magen Avraham, Taz, Shach, S'ma, Beis Shmuel, and Chelkas Mechokek are the major commentaries on the *Shulchan Aruch*.

Rema (glosses to the *Shulchan Aruch*) – Rabbi Moshe Isserles (Rema) was born around 1525 in Cracow, Poland. He was the rabbi of Cracow and an outstanding halachic authority. He appended important notes (*hagahos*) on Rabbi Yosef Karo's *Shulchan Aruch* that reflected Ashkenazic halachic practice. He also authored responsa and works about philosophy and kabbalah.

Nodah BeYehudah – Rabbi Yechezkel Landau was born in 1713 in Opataw, Poland, and passed away in 1793. In 1755, he became Chief Rabbi of Prague and all of Bohemia. He was one of the leaders of European Jewry during that time period. His famous responsa collection, *Nodah BeYehudah*, is considered a classic and authoritative work.

Mishnah Berurah – Rabbi Yisrael Meir HaKohen Kagan was born in 1839 and passed away in 1933. He lived in Radin, then Poland, now Belorussia. He established a yeshivah in Radin that ultimately became one of the most famous in Lithuania. His first halachic work was *Chafetz Chaim*, which dealt with the laws of *lashon hara*. His magnum opus was the *Mishnah Berurah* on the Orach Chaim section of *Shulchan Aruch*, in six volumes, which he spent twenty-eight years preparing (Warsaw 1884–Pietrkow 1907). This work consists of three parts: the *Mishnah Berurah* itself, which explains the *Shulchan Aruch*; Biur Halachah, which includes more detailed halachic discussions; and Sha'ar HaTziyun, which cites the sources of the rulings in the *Mishnah Berurah*.

Aruch HaShulchan – Rabbi Yechiel Michel HaLevi Epstein was born in 1829 in Bobroisk, Russia, and passed away in 1908. He was appointed rabbi of Novardok (Novogrodok), and headed the yeshivah there. He was one of the great Lithuanian halachic authorities. In the *Aruch HaShulchan*, he traces each halachah to its source, clarifies the differing opinions, and often explains the common practice and addresses many new halachic issues that arose in his times.

Igros Moshe – Rabbi Moshe Feinstein was born in Russia in 1895, and passed away in 1986. He served as rabbi in Luban, Russia, until he moved to the U.S. in 1937. He then became *rosh yeshivah* of Mesivta Tifereth Jerusalem in New York. He was the leading halachic authority of American Jewry, and his responsa deal with many modern issues. Rabbi Feinstein was active in Agudath Israel of America and Torah U'mesorah.

Minchas Shlomo – Rabbi Shlomo Zalman Auerbach was born in Jerusalem in 1910 and passed away in 1995. At age 22, he published a book titled *Meorei Aish* that dealt with the problems of electricity and Shabbos. Later, he became *rosh yeshivah* of Yeshivas Kol Torah. Many of his decisions and works related to the halachic problems that arose with modern technology.

Shevet HaLevi – Rabbi Shmuel HaLevi Wosner was born in Vienna, Austria, in 1914. He studied in Yeshivas Chachmei Lublin, where he became one of the close students of Rabbi Meir Shapiro. On the advice of the Chazon Ish, he was appointed rabbi of the Zichron Meir section of Bnei Brak, where he established Yeshivas Chachmei Lublin, and headed it until his recent passing.

Yabia Omer – Rabbi Ovadia Yosef was born in Baghdad in 1920 and passed away in 2013. In 1950, he served as rabbi of Tel Aviv, and later as the Sephardic Chief Rabbi of Israel, considered a world leader of Sephardic Jewry. The phenomenal breadth of his knowledge gives his responsa an encyclopedic quality. He also wrote *Yechaveh Da'as* and other works.

Tzitz Eliezer – Rabbi Eliezer Yehudah Waldenberg was born in 1916 in Jerusalem and passed away in 2006. He was Rabbi of Shaarei Zedek Medical Center in Jerusalem and was the head of a rabbinical court in Jerusalem. In 1945 he began to publish the twenty-two volumes of his responsa, entitled *Tzitz Eliezer* (the last volume was published in 1998). His responsa deal with all aspects of Jewish Law, in particular medical issues.

ABOUT THE AUTHOR

Rabbi Micha Cohn is a halachah writer for the Business Halachah Institute, and a *maggid shiur* at Yeshivah Meor HaTalmud. Rabbi Cohn founded the *Medical Halachah Email for Professionals* in 2011 to explore halachic issues in medicine and mental health. Currently, it has a readership of hundreds of observant medical and mental health professionals from around the world. Rabbi Cohn studied in Beth Medrash Govoha and Mesivta Tifereth Jerusalem, and interned at the Beis Hora'ah of Karlsberg and Beis Din of Philadelphia. He received *semichah* from Rabbi Shraga Feivel Zimmerman, presently Av Beis Din of Gateshead, England, and from Rabbi Ahron Felder, *zt"l*, of the Beis Din of Philadelphia.

לעילוי נשמות הורינו וזקנינו

ר׳ ישראל ז״ל ב״ר מאיר הי״ד

נלב״ע כה תמוז תשע״ג

וזוגתו

מרת צפורה ע״ה בת ר׳ נתן נטע ז״ל

נבל״ע כ״ב אדר תשע״ה

שטארק

In memory of our grandparents

Marian and Richard Lowenstein

רפאל בן אברהם ז״ל ושיינשין בת אורי ע״ה

DEDICATED BY ROBBY AND MASHA LOWENSTEIN

In memory of our grandparents

Bernie and Ruthie Tepper

ר' דוב ב"ר שלמה זלמן ז"ל

מרת רבקה לאה בת חיים ירוחם דוב ע"ה

לעילוי נשמת אמי מורתי

האשה החשובה שינדל ע"ה

בת ר' נחום דוב (פישביין) ז"ל

אשת חבר לא"מ

הרב יעקב שלמה מרדכי שליט"א

פינקלשטיין

נפטרה ביום ט' באב תשע"ד

ודודי

איש תם וישר וירא אלקים

הרב אברהם ברוך בהר"ר נחום דוב
ומרים דבורה פישביין ז"ל

נפטר ביום ח' כסלו תשע"ד

הרב יצחק זאב פינקלשטיין

לעילוי נשמת

בלימע פייגע בת אברהם ע"ה

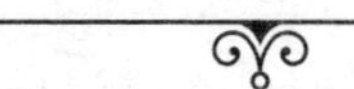

L'iluy Nishmas Our Parents

Millman ישראל בן יעקב ז"ל ונחמה לאה בת יהושע ע"ה

Hausman רחל בת אברהם ע"ה

Wishing continued *brachah* and *hatzlachah* to the esteemed author,
whom we are privileged to know

SHMUEL AND DEVORA MILLMAN, BOSTON

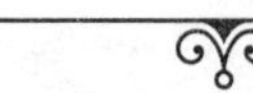

לעילוי נשמות הורינו

ר' שלמה בן יואל ז"ל וזוגתו מרת לאה בת מאיר ע"ה

ר' יצחק מאיר בן אליהו ז"ל וזוגתו מרת שרה בת זעליג ע"ה

הרב אליהו ואסתר מלכה פריד

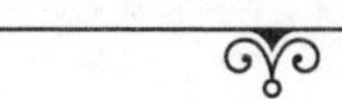

Dr. Howard Lebowitz
and the Specialty Hospital of Central New Jersey,
in appreciation of the Torah wisdom and guidance of Rabbi Micha Cohn

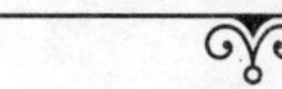

לעילוי נשמת זקנינו

מוהר"ר יקותיאל יהודה ב"ר אלכסנדר משה ז"ל

וזוגתו מרת ברכה ב"ר יוחנן ע"ה

הרה"ח ר' משה זאב ב"ר דוד ז"ל

וזוגתו מרת רחל ב"ר שמעיהו ע"ה

תנצב"ה

לעילוי נשמת הורינו וזקנינו
ר׳ יעקב ליב בן יחיאל ז״ל
ומרת יהודית בת מיכה ע״ה
ר׳ מרדכי ליב בן אברהם יעקב ז״ל

משפחת כהן

In Honor of
Rabbi Dovid and Mrs. Chaya Sara Cohn

DRS. YAAKOV AND SANDRA WEINREB

לעילוי נשמת אבי
ר׳ יעקב משה בן אברהם ז״ל

לע״נ
ר׳ יצחק בן גרשון שמריהו ז״ל

לע״נ
ר׳ צבי בן יואל ז״ל
ר׳ בנציון בן נחמיה הלוי ז״ל
אסתר בת משה הלוי ע״ה
פריידא בלימא בת מרדכי דוד ע״ה

לע״נ
ר׳ צבי בן משה יעקב ז״ל
מרים בת מרדכי ע״ה
ר׳ גדליהו בן שמעון ז״ל
חיה בת אריה ע״ה
אפרים ז״ל ב״ר חיים משה יוסף נ״י